ORDINARY WOMEN,
EXTRAORDINARY SEX

ORDINARY WOMEN, EXTRAORDINARY SEX

Every Woman's Guide to Pleasure and Beyond

by Dr. Sandra Scantling and Sue Browder

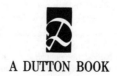

A DUTTON BOOK

DUTTON
Published by the Penguin Group
Penguin Books USA Inc., 375 Hudson Street,
New York, New York 10014, U.S.A.
Penguin Books Ltd, 27 Wrights Lane,
London W8 5TZ, England
Penguin Books Australia Ltd, Ringwood,
Victoria, Australia
Penguin Books Canada Ltd, 10 Alcorn Avenue,
Toronto, Ontario, Canada M4V 3B2
Penguin Books (N.Z.) Ltd, 182–190 Wairau Road,
Auckland 10, New Zealand

Penguin Books Ltd, Registered Offices:
Harmondsworth, Middlesex, England

First published by Dutton, an imprint of Dutton Signet,
a division of Penguin Books USA Inc.
Distributed in Canada by McClelland & Stewart Inc.

First Printing, October, 1993
10 9 8 7 6 5 4 3 2 1

Portions of this book were excerpted by *New Woman.*

The Absorption scale reproduced by permission from the Multidimensional Personality
Questionnaire copyright © 1978, 1982 by Auke Tellegen, publication forthcoming from the
University of Minnesota Press.

 REGISTERED TRADEMARK—MARCA REGISTRADA

LIBRARY OF CONGRESS CATALOGING IN PUBLICATION DATA:
Scantling, Sandra.
    Ordinary women, extraordinary sex : every woman's guide to pleasure and beyond /
by Sandra Scantling and Sue Browder.
        p.   cm.
    ISBN 0-525-93640-8
    1. Sex instruction for women. 2. Women—Sexual behavior. 3. Female orgasm. 4. Sex
(Psychology) I. Browder, Sue.
    II. Title.
HQ46.S336   1993
306.7'082—dc20   93–14562
                                                                      CIP

Printed in the United States of America
Set in Century Old Style

The cases presented herein are all real and are not composites. The names and identifying
details of the women and men discussed have been changed to protect their anonymity.

To Robert—My lover, critic, and best friend.
To my daughter, Jennifer—who is just beginning to discover
her extraordinary potential.
And to the memory of my brother—Stephan Neal Wolfe.
S.R.S

To Jennifer and Dustin,
who already know what holds a good marriage together.
S.E.B.

ACKNOWLEDGMENTS

I have been especially fortunate to have more than my share of outstanding teachers, mentors, and friends. To each of them, I extend my heartfelt gratitude: the late Dr. Elvin Semrad, for starting me on my journey of self-discovery. It was an honor and privilege to have been his supervisee. Annie Hargreaves, my first mentor at Boston University, for practicing what she preached about empathy; Dr. Sue M. Bishop, a remarkable woman and outstanding role model, for teaching me the true art of listening—to open my eyes, mind, and heart to my patients; Dr. Eugene Levitt, at Indiana University, for his expertise in sexual research; Dr. Paul Watzlawick, for his insights on reframing problems and turning them into solutions; Dr. Philip and Mrs. Lorna Sarrel at Yale University, for their years of sex therapy training and supervision, and for their continued friendship; Dr. Sidney Blatt and Dr. K. David Schultz at Yale University, for their expert clinical direction during my psychology fellowship; Dr.

Roger Peterson and Dr. David Singer, my doctoral mentors at Antioch New England Graduate School, for expecting clinical excellence from me by exemplifying it; Dr. Harry Fiss, a gifted supervisor and dear friend, for believing in me and staying in my corner for almost two decades; Dr. Natalie Lurie, my other "mother," confidante, and wise colleague—all wrapped into one, for her unfailing support; Ms. Claire E. O'Neil, former Assistant Hospital Director at the University of Connecticut Health Center, for encouraging me to persevere; Dr. Anthony Voytavich, teacher, friend, and physician par excellence at the University of Connecticut School of Medicine; Dr. Stephen Bank and Dr. Don Hiebel, for two enriching post doctoral years; Dr. John Money, for teaching me about Lovemaps; Guru Maharaj-Ji, for showing me that the source of all love and knowledge is inside of us.

There is one scientist whose suggestions and support were critical to my earlier research on absorption and to this book: Dr. Auke Tellegen. I am especially grateful to him for generously sharing his ideas, abundant time, and thought-provoking research. I would also like to recognize Dr. Don Mosher, for his sexual involvement theory; and Dr. Ulrich Neisser, for his valuable perspective on cognition, attention, and perception.

The research for this book could never have been completed without the assistance of the following: Dr. Lauren Hafner, for his statistical expertise; Gurujohn S. Khalsa and Gurujohn K. Khalsa, for distributing and collecting hundreds of questionnaires; St. Joseph College faculty, staff, and students; Kari Walker, the students, and staff of Central Connecticut State University; the professionals and staff who volunteered from Baystate Medical Center; Joan Handler, my friend and literary critic; and the many other individuals and agencies that participated in this study.

And a special thank-you to Ms. Deidre Elloian, for her invaluable computer wizardry during my final hours of need.

And to my family: my parents, Mr. and Mrs. Joseph Wolfe, for encouraging me to be a survivor; my children, Jennifer and Jesse, the loves of my life; and my husband, Robert Cooperman, for being by my side every step of this journey, offering his clinical wisdom, magical back rubs, and abundant love.

There is one individual who was pivotal to this project and my mainstay: Carole DeSanti, executive editor at Dutton. She believed in this book and its message from the start. I thank her for extending herself above and beyond the call of duty. Also to Julia Moskin, associate manuscript editor, for her many efforts and long hours at the fax machine.

Finally, my profound appreciation to all of the women and their partners who shared themselves and their super-sexual stories so candidly. Without their voices, this book would have been only a theory.

S.R.S.

I would like to thank a number of people who have influenced my thinking over the years and thus have helped make this book possible, including University of Connecticut professors Evelyn B. Thoman and Victor Denenberg; writer George Leonard, for launching my exploration of systems theory; and the late Carl Rogers, who was always generous with his interview time. Other scientists I would like to thank are Dr. Paul Byers at Columbia University, Dr. Mihaly Csikszentmihalyi at the University of Chicago, Dr. Julian Davidson of Stanford University, and University of West Florida psychologist Gayle Privette, Ph.D., for sharing their research and expertise.

In addition, I would like to extend a special thanks to literary agent Geri Thoma, who understood the book from the beginning and offered countless valuable insights; editor Carole DeSanti, for her unflagging enthusiasm and support even when the going got rough; my dear friend and longtime editor and colleague Donna Jackson, whose advice was always wisely on target; Liz O'Neil, who was there for me night and day; my daughter Erin Browder and son Dustin Browder, for their hours of arduous transcription; Jennifer Brock, for her tireless library research; the production staff at Dutton for their patience and efficiency; and most of all, my husband and best friend Walter, for his unceasing support, courage, and understanding.

S.E.B.

CONTENTS

Prologue   xiii

Part I: SUPERSEXUAL EXPERIENCE DESCRIBED

1. Going Beyond All Sexual Boundaries   3
2. Others Who Found It   19
3. Women Describe Their Most
   Passionate Moments   31
4. Dissecting the Rose   45
5. Supersex, Peak Peformance, and Flow   55
6. Supersex and Beyond: Bringing Passion
   to All Experience   69
7. What's the Partner's Role?   79
8. Courageously Opening to Life   93

xi

Part II: BECOMING SUPERSEXUAL

9. Those Who Learn Young   107

10. Those Who Learn Later in Life   117

11. Finding Your Absorption Style   135

12. The Supersexual Mind-Set   185

13. Building Your Ecstasy Connection   209

Appendix: Guided Imagery   221

Bibliography   227

Authors' Note   239

Index   241

PROLOGUE

The human mind, once stretched to a new idea,
never goes back to its original dimensions.

—Oliver Wendell Holmes

What is it that makes sexual experience so passionate? What are the keys to sexual arousal? Why is one sexual moment a turn-off and another seemingly similar time a tremendous turn-on? Does enjoyment of peak sex depend on your partner, the setting, your frame of mind, or something else?

These are the questions I began to ask in my sex therapy practice more than twenty years ago. As I treated thousands of individuals and couples with a wide range of problems, a number of interesting patterns emerged. Some women described having problems with sexual desire, arousal, or response with one partner and not with another; or with the same partner on one occasion and not on another. But others—whom I came to think of as "pleasure experts"—experienced such intense passion during intimate moments that many of them reported feeling as if they were floating in space, seeing spectacular displays of light ("liquid fireworks," as one woman put it), being charged with electricity, or being transported to other places. They revealed that at times they could feel turned on or experience orgasm with "no touch at all," just through their thinking and imagination. These women reported an ability to "get lost" in their arousal and described feelings of ecstasy and an ultimate connection beyond words—beyond orgasm—beyond sexual pleasure as it has been conventionally defined. And they returned from these experiences with renewed energy, creativity, and lust for life.

I became fascinated with and inspired by these women. If we could identify the keys to what I came to think of as "supersexual" connections, perhaps we could use this information to enhance pleasure for *all* of us. Who were these "supersexual" women? How did they come to have such extraordinary sexual experiences? Is the capacity for peak sex a personality trait that some "lucky" individuals are born with, or is it something that we can all experience? If it is a personality trait, what trait is it? I wanted to discover as much as possible about the actual ingredients of these sexual encounters and the women who were able to reach beyond sexual limits.

My first encounter with a "pleasure expert" was in 1972. The early seventies were exciting times for psychological growth-enhancing opportunities. T-groups ("T" for training) or "encounter groups" at the National Training Laboratories in Bethel, Maine, were led by nontraditionalists who were experimenting with creative alternatives to psychological change. The Esalen-based human potential movement at Big Sur in California was in full force. It was a time of mind expansion and, for many, a time of increased self-awareness and responsibility.

I met Mary while attending a Will Schutz workshop at Esalen. Schutz had written the book *Joy* in 1967. His background included psychodrama, bioenergetics, and Gestalt therapy. Schutz writes, "If there is one statement true of every living person it must be this: I haven't yet reached my full potential." He believes that joy is the feeling that comes from the fulfillment of potential.

Mary seemed to exude pure joy. I wondered if she also felt a special joy in sexual moments and decided to ask her. Mary was my first teacher on this subject. She was a woman in her late fifties who welcomed passion with all of her being. We spoke for hours as I became more and more interested in identifying her talent for living passionately. Mary described life as a river and said that many people are afraid that they will get swept up in the current, so they either stand timidly on the banks, or they enter the water and go "against the flow." Swimming upstream inevitably leads to exhaustion, frustration, and a general disappointment in the journey. Mary had learned to "go with the flow" in her life and enjoy the feeling of being in the current, but she had also learned to steer around the rocks.

Mary had discovered what we labeled as her "pleasure profile." She seemed to be in touch with myriad senses, thoughts, feelings, images—both conscious and beyond conscious awareness—that brought her intense joy. She was also able to transfer this insight from nonsexual moments to explicitly sexual times, whether alone or with a partner.

Through the years when we were friends, Mary introduced me to Barry Steven's book *Don't Push the River (It Flows By Itself)*, and to her experiences with Zen, meditation, and the teachings of Krishnamurti. I remember her saying that she had discovered the ways she confused herself by dwelling in what Krishnamurti called "the shallow mind" and that there were many thoughts—all kinds of thoughts—that had once blocked her from feeling pleasure. External concerns and pressures competed with her appreciation of the beauty inside herself, the beauty that was always there. The "shallow mind" thinks thoughts that don't come *from you,* yet you have come to think of it *as you.* Krishnamurti says, "Right thinking is essential for right living." But what is "right" thinking? He teaches that it is an inner experience of self-knowledge that reflects the true essence of the self—one's passions and joys. It is not blind conformity to a pattern set by society or the mere reaction against such a pattern. Right thinking is not a *thing* to be achieved, it is an experience to be lived.

At the time I met Mary, I was on the faculty of Indiana-Purdue University while completing my graduate studies. Dr. Eugene Levitt, Chairman of the Department of Psychology and an expert in research on sexuality, was one of my thesis advisors. His guidance, along with the supervision of Dr. Sue Bishop and many others, stimulated my clinical interest in sex-related issues. There was so much to learn—so many sexual frontiers waiting to be explored.

In the early seventies, the field of sexuality as a whole was relatively young—the ground-breaking research of William Masters and Virginia Johnson had only recently been completed. By observing thousands of sex response cycles in hundreds of men and women, Masters and Johnson identified and described the physiological phases of the sex response cycle and the similarities and differences in sexual response. Beyond this knowledge of physiological functioning and that of sexual practices contributed by Alfred Kinsey in 1948 and 1953, the vast world of psychological issues was waiting to be explored. Dysfunctional sexuality had begun to be addressed, and terms like *performance anxiety, spectatoring,* and *goal orientation* emerged in the literature.

But what about peak sex or what I came to think of as "supersexual" experience? How could we learn more about the keys to healthy, highly pleasurable sexuality? I determined to approach the subject from the inside-out, not from the outside-in, and to learn more specifically about arousal by listening to women and their descriptions of extraordinary sexual experiences.

In the years that followed, I completed advanced training in sex therapy at Yale University under the direction of Dr. Phil and Mrs. Lorna Sarrel, earned a doctorate in clinical psychology, and received a psychology fellowship at Yale. I became a certified sex therapist and continued to interview and treat hundreds of women and couples— paying attention to what makes sex especially pleasurable. It became apparent that my speculation of many years before was true: that women who were "pleasure experts"— experiencing the heights of sexual pleasure—had access to a different kind of reality, a reality that opens us to opportunities for wonder, excitement, and joy in things that often go unnoticed. I sensed that although these women were perfectly "ordinary women" like you or me, they were also "supersexual," and had discovered something of profound value about the enjoyment of sexuality that they could teach all women.

But what was it specifically that led women to experience peak sex? Could it really be that some combination of the readiness to see things differently and the ability to absorb fully in a moment were the keys to experiencing passion that knows no limits? My inquiry into these questions broadened and deepened, and my doctoral research was structured around these questions. Two important, scientifically valid findings emerged. First, the *best* predictor of intense sexual pleasure was the women's ability to become fully absorbed in the moment; and second, their enjoyment of imagery, fantasy, and daydreaming (which seemed to go hand in hand with absorption) was also associated with peak sexual arousal. But what was perhaps most exciting was what I discovered serendipitously after completing the "formal" aspects of my research.

During the "exit interviews," when participants are generally "debriefed," many of the women described what we now call "supersexual" experiences. Some of them reported being "lost in the imagery," "unaware of time or place," and one person described a feeling of "floating" above her body. What was really going on here? Were the women who described being lost in imagery and reporting peak arousal unusual or atypical in some dysfunctional sense—or was there a phenomenon here that many women experience but may not have the words or opportunity to fully describe? Although it has often been said that the mind is the most powerful organ of sexual pleasure, what is *really* meant by saying that the locus of enjoyment is in the mind? All of these questions deserved a much closer look.

Writer Sue Browder and I met in 1978. From the very first conversation there was a remarkable synergy between us. A few years ago, when I shared my research about supersexual response with her, she expressed excitement about the potential for enhancing women's sexual pleasure. Together we explored the journeys our pleasure experts have taken to their extraordinary supersexual experiences.

The 86 women studied for this book were selected from 536 women who completed a scientifically well-validated measure of "absorption" developed by psychologist Auke Tellegen. The Tellegen scale, which is not sexual in nature, consistently and reliably identified the women who were "high absorbers"—women who had "an openness to absorbing and self-altering experiences." I predicted that these were the same women who were most likely to have "supersex." The prediction proved correct.

The population studied came from college dormitories,

yoga classes, retirement communities, theaters for the deaf, professional organizations, and word-of-mouth networks. Although men were not the focus of the study, we did interview some of the partners of our "supersexual" women in an effort to better understand their relationships.

After completing the initial screening, a group of sixty-eight "high absorbers" and eighteen "low absorbers" were studied further. Each of these women completed the 300-item Tellegen Multidimensional Personality Inventory, a demographic questionnaire, and an in-depth audiotaped interview which was later transcribed and analyzed for various themes and patterns. *Ordinary Women, Extraordinary Sex* presents the results of this research and the many voices of the women studied.

It is important to mention here that these are *ordinary* women who experience moments of deep absorption. These episodes are similar to what happens to all of us when we daydream or our mind "wanders"—one part of our consciousness gets suspended or separated from another. These are *not* women who have a split in their personality structure or report prolonged periods of amnesia, as is the case in the diagnoses of multiple personality disorder or other psychiatric conditions. Because these are ordinary women, we feel more confident in our ability to generalize from our findings.

The women are not formally (or uniformly) involved in nontraditional sexual (e.g., Tantric) or meditational practices. From all that they have said or displayed, they appear to be "normal," physically and mentally healthy women. But they have experienced pleasure and pain and have learned to adapt to many of life's challenges—including sexual learning—in creative and special ways.

Our "pleasure experts" include single and married women; heterosexual, lesbian, and bisexual women; young, middle-aged, and older women; nature-lovers and urbanites. Some are hard-driving professionals; others are fully satisfied stay-at-home mothers. These are women whose mind-body-spirit connection comes through their enjoyment of and full absorption in everyday events, in a special attitude toward life itself.

What does this say about the journey to sexual ecstasy? It tells us that there are many pathways to this experience. Every one of you reading this book has everything necessary to have this experience for yourself. Nothing is missing. If you can recall a moment of pleasure in your life, you have proof that you have tasted this experience and can learn to drink more deeply. You already have all that you need inside you, but you may not have known where to look, or how to identify the treasures within.

In the following chapters, you'll share in our discovery of supersexual joy and in your own potential, through the voices of the women who have in many ways become our teachers.

Dr. Sandra R. Scantling
Farmington, Connecticut
1993

We have it in us to be splendid.
—Maya Angelou

∞ PART I ∞

Supersexual
Experience Described

CHAPTER 1

Going Beyond All Sexual Boundaries

The information in any real situation is indefinitely rich. There is always more to see than anyone sees, and more to know than anyone knows.

—psychologist Ulrich Neisser,
Cognition and Reality

Catherine is thirty-nine and works as a court stenographer. She is an intelligent, forthright person with a passion for life, and until recently, she was having ordinary, pleasurable, genital-focused orgasms with her lover. But about two years ago, she began having a different kind of sexual experience—one so unbelievably intense she was taken beyond all previous sexual boundaries.

She describes one of her most memorable episodes this way:

I was lying in the living room on my queen-sized sofa bed, sipping bordeaux and listening to a Van Morrison tape. It was a cool evening and light from the full moon was streaming through the lace curtains from a large window near the bed. I'd also lit some candles. It was a very romantic setting, but nothing felt contrived. I was doing all this for myself because it felt so good, not to "set the scene for sex," if you know what I mean. I was looking forward to

3

him being there, but not necessarily in a sexual way. I was just anticipating spending some time with him. I was feeling very languid, very relaxed.

Suddenly, he walked in and there was just this incredible electricity between us. We didn't even say a word. He simply came over, lay down beside me, and we just took *off!* I instantly felt a sense of totally letting go, but not being afraid of losing control. It was like I was flying.

I always feel completely trusting of him. I'm never afraid he will do anything to hurt me or anything bad will happen when I'm with him. I feel very safe. As we made love, he told me how happy he was to be with me, how much he'd missed me that day. And I knew he wasn't just saying those things because he liked making love. His feelings were sincere and had specifically to do with *me*. But it didn't just have to do with me, it had everything to do with the *two* of us. There was an incredible sense of connectedness. Everything felt absolutely right.

I don't know how long we made love. I think maybe it was about three hours. We sometimes make love for as long as eight hours straight. We often feel as if we could go on and on and on. What amazes me most is the way *he* can go on and on. He often jokes about it, saying, "You know this is impossible. We're defying the laws of physics. But it's happening." But he says he's never been able to do this with anyone else. It's because of me, because of the way we are together. We're just so in tune with each other. I remember as we made love that night thinking how much I love him and how much he loves me, how much we mean to each other.

At one point, I just transcended the physical. It was like everything was involved: my mind, my body, my whole spiritual being. [She laughs lightly, joyously.] That's when I thought I saw God. What did God look like? [long pause] White. There was just all this amazing light, very bright but not the least stark. In fact, this light was soft—almost like a cloud. I remember feeling a sensation of not being physically there anymore, just floating in that bright, safe, peaceful light. I must have had an orgasm at that point, but this feeling was *beyond* orgasm. It was a feeling of spiritual connection so deep I can't even describe it. I don't know how much time passed. But I slowly became aware of lying there on the sofa bed beside him. I remember thinking, "This is the way it's supposed to be. This is what they mean when they talk about seeing fireworks and hearing angels singing."

The ecstasy Catherine felt that night in the moonlight goes far beyond what we've come to think of as sex or sexual pleasure. Catherine says this particular experience, in which she transcended physical sensations and felt wholly connected, left her psychologically stronger: "I just have much more awareness of myself. I feel more complete as a person in ways it's hard to explain. I'm more aware of what I'm capable of feeling and experiencing. I've come to realize there's not just a needy little girl inside me who needs to be nurtured, but there's an independent, grown *woman* in me who needs nurturing, too, and that's not a sign of weakness—that's okay." She adds, "It's like my spiritual and sexual selves aren't separate anymore. I've acquired a much greater sense of wholeness and inner peace."

A forty-two-year-old executive with an engaging smile and short salt-and-pepper hair, Debra exudes an air of self-confidence, determination, and independence. She dresses professionally and conservatively, but with her own personal flair. At thirty-seven, Debra had recently left a stifling marriage and decided to have sex one night with a man about ten years her junior who had been pursuing her. She describes what happened:

The whole evening went perfectly from start to finish. He came over to my house, we ate by candlelight and cuddled and kissed on the couch. Then he carried me up to my bedroom. You know, the Rhett Butler kind of scenario. I'd never made love with a man so verbal during sex, and I just loved that. It was a real turn-on for me ... right in the middle of lovemaking he sat straight up in bed and shouted, "Holy shit! This is so much fun!" I loved that. It was just so refreshing and honest. I didn't have to worry about whether or not he was having a good time because I *knew* he was. So I could totally concentrate on myself. I'm usually a person who always has to be in control, but I lost all control. It was total sexual abandon. I wasn't aware of him, me, or the room. I was just lost in the moment. That night, I had what I called at the time a "mind orgasm." It wasn't just a physical sensation, it was a real spiritual event. I had no conception of time and space. It felt like I was in a time warp. I was totally nowhere. I'd had sex all my adult life. But this was the first time I experienced what lovemaking is all about.

Debra says that experiencing this single "mind orgasm"—which she also calls a "spiritual orgasm"—changed her forever. "It renewed my sexuality, my confidence, and my zest for life," she explains. "It also helped me see my sexuality as my own. I discovered for the first time that I could have sex for *me,* for *my* pleasure, and I didn't always have to be worrying about whether or not the man was having a good time."

During one of these experiences, a woman goes beyond what she has believed possible sexually. "I saw and felt an intense arousal—as if the universe stood still," recalls Claire, fifty-two, who owns a small business and has been married and divorced twice. "Everything felt connected—my body, my feelings, my spirit—in one harmonious whole. There were no boundaries, only connections within myself and between me and the man I was with. . . . I was totally unaware of anything else."

Catherine, Debra, and Claire, along with a selected group of "high absorbers" identified from a population of five hundred and thirty-six women—reported imagery during sex that approaches the sublime. They spoke of sex as it "should" be—the way we always thought it could be—the way it is not for the majority of women. We found women who hear music, smell the ocean air, feel as if they're flying and see flashing lights, sparks, swirling colors, and stars. These visions and images come to them unbidden—like delightful gifts from another dimension. "Right before orgasm I saw blues and purples. It wasn't like this Crayola color ... it was more like a flash," says Margaret, thirty-eight, who began reaching supersexual ecstasy during her second marriage. Megan, forty, who connects supersexually with her husband of two years, says, "Usually during or right after orgasm, I see very soft colors: pinks, peaches, delicate greens. I also sometimes hear sounds—like the ocean waves or the wind rushing through the trees." A third woman reports: "You know in *Star Wars* where Luke Skywalker and Han Solo go into warp speed and all of a sudden—whoosh!—the stars just elongate? It was like that. It was like shooting out to the stars."

At these moments, a woman transcends all self-consciousness and self-judgment. Everything seems "just right." Free from doubts, inhibitions, and controls, she feels at her most spontaneous, alert, and creative. She concentrates without trying to concentrate. No longer striving, needing, or wishing for anything other than what she has, she just *is*. And when she feels such intense joy that she loses all awareness of time and her surroundings, she feels fortunate, "graced." Asked if she thinks she could have enjoyed this level of sexual response earlier in her life, Debra replies, "I don't know. I didn't question that. I just felt blessed that it had happened."

Philosopher William James suggested more than a century ago that the best way to understand religion would be to study the most religious man during his most ardent religious moments. Similarly, we theorized that to unlock the deepest mysteries of female sexuality, we needed to study the most sexually responsive women during their most passionate sexual encounters.

You might picture human sexual pleasure as lying on a continuum of pleasure, with unsatisfying sex at one end of the scale and the ecstatic experiences these women describe at the other.

At the low-pleasure end of the scale lies unsatisfying sex, which includes a wide range of problems. Among them: feeling little or no desire; having pain during sex; an inability to get or stay turned on, to discuss sexual problems with one's partner, or to experience orgasm if one wants to. At this end of the scale, a woman is paying attention during sex to what we might call "shoulds" and "oughts"—voices that distract her and block pleasure.

In the middle of the scale lies "satisfying" sex. When operating in this range of the scale, you usually feel comfortable and connected with your partner. Most of the time, you may feel that nothing is missing. You have accurate sexual information, can talk with your partner about most sexual concerns, and find you make love as often as you wish and respond in a way that satisfies you. During sex, your mind stays focused on physical sensations, specific body parts, or your relationship.

At the uppermost end of the pleasure scale—the point women like Catherine and Debra have reached—you're going far beyond ordinary sex. You begin by focusing on specific sensations and allow your sexual pleasure to take you to another dimension of pleasure.

Since no word has ever been used to describe the ineffable joy at this end of the scale, we struggled with what to call this experience. "Bliss" seemed too tame. "Rapture" contained the sense of being overwhelmed by emotion.

These women were certainly in "ecstasy," but many people had already used that word to describe ordinary sex. After much thought, we finally decided to call these experiences *supersex,* from the prefix *super-,* meaning "over and above, exceeding the norm, or surpassing all others of its kind." Supersexual experience involves extraordinary bliss and altered states of consciousness. In this state, you're going beyond orgasm to experience an ecstatic mind-body-spirit connection. After even one of these experiences, many women report feeling psychologically "healed" or transformed. There is as much difference between ordinary sex and supersex as there is between physics and metaphysics.

Here, then, is how we envision the spectrum of sexual pleasure:

A_____B_____C....................
Unsatisfying Sex Satisfying Sex   Supersex
(low pleasure)   (doing okay)   (peak pleasure and beyond)

The vast majority of sexual solutions and guidance over the past five decades has been drawn from studies of people operating in the "A to B" range on the scale. Along the continuum from B to C—and especially at the "supersexual" end of the scale—research has been very limited. In this research we set out to explore the "B to C" segment of the scale, focusing specifically on women who had reached point C in their journey—the ultimate in sexual fulfillment and joy. "Point C" is infinite, since the potential to deepen sexual joy is limitless.

So how did we find these women? Obviously, we couldn't simply ask women if they were having great sex because each woman will define "great" differently. One woman may think it's terrific if she enjoys an orgasm every fourth time she makes love; another may enjoy three orgasms a night and still feel something is missing. We could have asked women if they were easily orgasmic, then interviewed those who said yes. But this approach, used several times in the past by other researchers, poses a major problem in that it assumes that intense sexual pleasure is measured only in terms of *orgasms,* when, in fact, orgasm is an insufficient measure of pleasure or satisfaction. So how could we locate women who had already reached "point C" on the pleasure scale?

One scientific tool helped locate supersexual women with amazing precision. This was the absorption scale developed by University of Minnesota psychologist Auke Tellegen. In a paper published in 1974, Dr. Tellegen described a thirty-four-question scale he had designed to measure "absorption," which he broadly defined as "an openness to absorbing and self-altering experiences." Simply put, absorption is the ability to become deeply immersed in any experience that intrigues you. Women who can become so immersed in sex that they lose all sense of time, self, and space turn out to be the *same* women who can become easily lost in a sunset, the rhythmic beat of reggae, the strains of a Mozart concerto, or work they love. Trusting their own perceptions and possessing the ability to make independent decisions about rules imposed by outside authorities, these women, whom we came to call "high absorbers," experience life in fresh, original ways. They are often greatly moved by poetic language, feel imaginatively stimulated by the crackle and flames of a wood fire, and take delight in such small pleasures as the five-pointed star shape you see when you cut an apple across the core. When listening to powerful music, such as an organ playing in church, many feel as if they're being lifted right up in the air or as if they're "riding" the music like a roller coaster. Many of these women also smell certain aromas when they see certain colors. One woman told us, for example, that when she sees red, she often smells cinnamon (in fact, she describes the color as "cinnamon-apple red"), and when she sees a certain shade of blue, she smells sea air.

Most important, the women we studied have intensely vivid imaginations. When they read a novel or watch a movie, they can get so lost in the story they "become one" with the characters. Long after a movie has ended, they can return to the story in their minds and relive it as if it were real. They can also travel to far-off places in their imaginations. Kimberly, twenty-two, says, "We went to Cabo San Lucas last year. And if I'm feeling bad, I can close my eyes and I'm back in Cabo. It's weird because I can be freezing cold, but when I close my eyes I'm back in Cabo: the sand is hot, my skin is glowing, and the water is warm and blue. Then when I open my eyes again, I feel better and I'm not cold anymore."

We tend to think that what we experience in life depends on the sights, sounds, tastes, textures, and smells that are "out there." But increasingly, we are beginning to understand that what you perceive "out there" depends on what you're inwardly *ready* to perceive. The high absorbing supersexual women we met are somehow more ready to see, smell, or feel the beauty in a rose or to appreciate a sunset. They have a special mind-set that allows them to appreciate the world around and inside them, and to enjoy sex in brand-new ways. In this book, we want to help you see yourself and your life through the mind-set with which supersexual women address the world.

Physically, the women interviewed for this book *look* quite ordinary. Although some are young and physically fit, the majority are over thirty-five and come in a variety of shapes and sizes. Two are deaf. Several are over sixty. They are college students, waitresses, homemakers, nurses, artists, attorneys, and yoga instructors. They are married, divorced, single and widowed, ages eighteen to sixty-three, with incomes of $5,000 to more than $150,000 a year. Their religions run the gamut, from Roman Catholic, Protestant, Jewish, and Buddhist to Sikh, Quaker, and undecided. They are Caucasian, African American, Asian, and Hispanic. Most are heterosexual, but some are bisexual and lesbian. A number of these women were sexually abused as children. One had a double mastectomy at age thirty. Some have overcome the trauma of being raped. Though not a representative sample of the entire population, the women in this book are an extremely diverse group from all walks of life.

If you were in a room with the women in this book, the first thing you'd notice is how distinctly individual they look. Rose, that Rubenesque woman in the Laura Ashley print skirt and yellow high-top sneakers, works in a bank and has been happily married for eight years to a caterer. The neatly dressed, plain-faced pregnant woman with just a touch of makeup is Mary Anne, a full-time mother, married twelve years. The redhead by the door—the one in her early twenties wearing a purple Danskin top and tight hip-hugging jeans—is Alex, a college student working part-time as a bartender. The middle-aged man standing beside her—the one about five feet, four inches tall and balding—is Joe, the man who can make love to Catherine for eight hours. Myra is a round-faced, silver-haired history professor in her mid-fifties with deep laugh lines at the corners of her blue eyes; Jacqueline, a thirty-five-year-old attorney with dark-rimmed glasses set on a slightly crooked nose, and hair pulled back in a chignon; Josephine, a thirty-six-year-old museum curator who weighs about 250 pounds and expresses her aesthetic sense by wearing feather earrings and an East Indian print skirt. Serena, forty-one, is six feet tall and moves with the grace of a dancer; and Darla, forty-one, has high cheekbones, is religious and homespun, wears chinos and sneakers, and looks as if she just came in from weeding her garden. The message: Forget the superficial dictates of magazines and movies. Women who enjoy extraordinary sex aren't doing so because they conform to artificial standards of female beauty or have especially handsome partners. This sexual experience has nothing to do with how you look. It has to do with the choices you make and how in touch with yourself you've become. What we found from studying these women is that when something—or someone—captures their interest, they have the remarkable ability to direct their attention to it and open themselves fully to the experience. They have the capacity to feel fully alive. Additionally, we found that for a high absorber, sex doesn't grow dull with the same partner year after year because when she touches or is touched by her lover, she often becomes so immersed in joy she feels as if she's making love for the first time.

Many questions arose as we began considering this phenomenon. One of the first was: Were these women born with this incredible gift, or did they learn it? Some of these women seem to have had a head start. Serena, a tall, elegant teacher who has been deaf from birth, described to us through an interpreter what happened to her when she was masturbating at age five:

> I'll always remember that experience because it shocked me so much. I felt my body start to control me, and I didn't know what was happening. I didn't feel ashamed or guilty, it was nothing like that. My mother had never talked to me about sex, so I figured it was just supposed to be natural. My body felt strangely exciting, and I was wondering why I was enjoying it. At first it just felt good. But then it went on and on and on, and I let go. Suddenly I felt myself separate from my body. I felt I wasn't in my body anymore. I

was *out* of body. It was very peaceful and pleasant. I was concentrating on this feeling of peace and the feeling of *traveling*—like I was traveling with the orgasm. I was a kid, but I felt like *more* than a kid. I felt very powerful.

Later she said this capability grew in her. By the time she was twenty, "I could have a powerful orgasm and see swirling colors just by looking in a mirror: I didn't even have to touch myself. Sometimes it was even beyond my control. It would just happen."

Yet even though a few women seem to recall supersexual feelings when they were quite young, this research confirms that the vast majority *learned* to reach supersexual peaks. We believe the ability to enjoy peak sex is an inborn capacity that is later developed by interacting with life experiences. Many of the women studied didn't report feeling supersexual pleasure until midlife or later, and a large number said that their first sexual intercourse was "average" or "disappointing." When asked to describe how pleasurable they found their first sexual intercourse on a scale of 0 (not at all enjoyable) to 6 (extremely enjoyable), the average response was a 3. This is not to equate supersexual passion with intercourse, but to note that sexual enjoyment can continue to unfold and deepen over the years.

As Debra observes: "I think it would be a rare woman who could have a peak sexual experience the first time. A woman needs to understand that what she feels when she experiences her own sexuality isn't all it's ever going to be. You have to cultivate sexuality, just like you have to cultivate a lot of good things in life, just as you must with your personality or your marriage."

"My first time was disappointing," recalls Lillian, a twenty-two-year-old waitress attending night school. "It didn't make me feel as physically, emotionally, and spiritually wonderful as I thought it would."

Some women believed their disappointment sprang from the fact that the man was "clumsy" or the mood was wrong. One woman believed her first intercourse was unpleasant because the setting was an unromantic motel room and she had always dreamed it would happen in a meadow or by a brook in the moonlight. Another rated her first intercourse as a 0 on the pleasure scale because "my partner was interested in getting, not giving pleasure."

But even Brett, a twenty-year-old college student who lost her virginity to a considerate, sensitive man, found her first time profoundly disappointing. "We had planned it, we knew we were going to do it, and that whole day I was a basket case," she recalls. "I was saying to myself, 'Oh, my God, I don't believe I'm going to do this.' I wanted to. I really wanted to. But I was scared. So we went for a walk on the golf course after dark and on the fourteenth hole he had a blanket spread out and a couple of candles. It was so romantic I just let it happen. I guess my nervousness prevented me from really enjoying it and intercourse was uncomfortable. The second time was better, but I was thinking, 'This is *it?*'"

A few women said the first time was great—or at least reasonably okay. "It was nice," recalls Mara, a twenty-seven-year-old journalist. "It wasn't like 'Wow! Great! Check it out!' But it was nice. I was completely ready for it. I decided I was in love with the man, and I went on the pill beforehand. So I made the decision ahead of time that I was going to do it, and it was like, 'Okay, I'm ready.'"

For many women, first intercourse is often less than magical. Here are some reasons given by our subjects:

- "I didn't know what I was doing. It was all too new and I was so inexperienced."
- "I was nervous."

- "It was too quick, and I didn't have time to get turned on or have an orgasm."
- "Penetration was painful, and I didn't tell him."
- "It felt too mechanical. I didn't know how I was supposed to feel."
- "I felt it was wrong, against everything I'd been taught. It's hard to relax when you feel that way!"
- "It was with a stranger, uncomfortable, no emotional attachment."
- "I wasn't emotionally ready, felt pressured and kind of used."
- "I was raped the first time—it left emotional scars."

For these women, somewhere between such disappointing or traumatic first sexual encounters and our interviews with them years later, sex became extraordinary. In short, these women are not simply lucky. They have actively influenced their experience of sexual pleasure. In reality, every one of us is already traveling the same road. Supersexual women—our real experts and teachers—have merely journeyed farther, opened further to pleasure, and can show us all more clearly how to find our own way.

Transcending Cultural Messages

Too often when a woman feels dissatisfied with some aspect of sex, she blames herself and/or her partner for being flawed in some way, when the problem may rest in her acceptance of the culture's messages about the way sex "should" or "ought to" be. The women in this book have transcended many cultural messages about what we "should" think, feel, and do to have intensely erotic experiences. Among these are some myths: that the best way to enliven one's sex life is to focus on changing some *thing* (finding a more exotic position, wearing sexy lingerie, losing ten pounds) instead of changing one's *perspective;* that the genitally focused orgasm is the ultimate "goal"; that when it comes to a woman's sexual fulfillment her partner's physical endowments matter more than a loving nature; that novelty in the situation or in one's partner (rather than discovering one's own special source for pleasure) is what most heightens excitement; or that others have more answers than a woman herself possesses within.

This is a different kind of self-help book. Our focus is on what you're already doing *right* and how you can enhance your pleasure even further. While sexual variation, erotic attire, and other novelties can certainly spice up sex, discovering your own special internal source of pleasure will create lasting freshness. In this book, you will discover how to empower yourself—to find that inner pleasure source and take full advantage of your potential for sexual joy. As the women in our study reveal, extraordinary sex comes to you naturally when you begin to discover how to open to pleasure, and to become more fully absorbed in what brings you joy.

∽ CHAPTER 2 ∽

Others Who Found It

*"It's like I'm in the center of the universe and I
see this great whirlpool of color—every color of
the rainbow—swirling like those pictures you
see of the stars swirling in the cosmos."*

On first hearing what's going through a woman's mind
during a true peak sexual moment—on hearing her speaking of "swirling blue sparks," "floating in a white cloud," or
"zooming into hyperspace"—those who have never had
this experience themselves might wonder whether these
women are describing orgasms or something else. This
leads us to ask a number of questions: Why hasn't anyone
noticed this phenomenon before now? If there's a whole-
body response more intense than an orgasm, why has orgasm been regarded for so long as the ultimate sexual
high?

Mostly because women haven't been talking about these
experiences. Why not? It could be because intense female
eroticism still remains taboo. But we think one explanation
is that these experiences are so elusive it is hard to find
words to describe them. Many of the women we spoke to
volunteered that they hadn't even told their lovers or best
friends about their supersexual experiences.

Georgia, a high-energy forty-three-year-old kindergarten teacher who has been married twenty-two years and has a warm love of people that draws others to her, says, "I tell my husband everything—how I'm feeling, why I'm worried, what I did all day, even what I had for lunch. But, you know, it's strange: I've never told him that during those times when our lovemaking is most intense, I often find myself swinging in an open-weave rope hammock between two big, leafy oak trees. The place is very shady, usually surrounded by the ocean, and the surf is pounding on the rocks. I'm just in that hammock all by myself, enjoying the breeze and the wonderful quiet. Then it's over and I'm back on the bed or the floor." If women don't even tell the people dearest to them about these incredible moments, is it any wonder they've seldom told sex researchers? A woman might tell a sex researcher she has orgasms. But if a researcher should ask a woman to recall the most intense sexual moment of her life, it's unlikely that she will casually volunteer that along with her intense physical arousal, she also sees blue sparks, feels herself swinging in a hammock, or smells sea air.

Supersex and Mysticism

That's not to say scientists have *never* recorded descriptions of profound sexual ecstasy. The experience we call supersex was uncovered by scientists at least as early as the 1960s. But it wasn't reported by sex researchers. It was described by scientists investigating mystical experiences. In *Ecstasy: A Study of Some Secular and Religious Experiences* (published in 1962 by Indiana University Press), researcher Margharita Laski reported that her extensive studies of mystical experiences revealed that sexual love was a common "trigger" for mystical ecstasy. Of the small sample of people she surveyed who were having mystical experiences, 43 percent (eighteen women and eight men) mentioned reaching peaks of ecstasy during sex. Looking at key words and phrases used to describe mystical moments, Laski found as we did that people described sexual ecstasy in much the same way they described becoming immersed in other pleasures, such as listening to music, reading a book, or viewing a painting. Among other sensations, they reported feelings of unity ("everything . . . falling into place"); timelessness ("sensation of timeless bliss—life should be like this forever"); overwhelming passion ("the emotion was strong enough to carry with it everything—reason, soul, blood—in a great sweep"); and a feeling of perfection ("it wasn't just sex, it was everything right at that moment . . . as if nothing could ever go wrong again"). During sexual ecstasy, women and men also reported "becoming airborne," floating, and flowing like liquid ("the hard lines . . . are gone . . . one flows over them"). All these perceptions were also reported by the women we studied.

Another scientist who found women and men pushing beyond the boundaries of conventional sexuality was University of Chicago sociologist and theologian Andrew M. Greeley. In *Ecstasy: A Way of Knowing,* written in the early seventies, Greeley wrote: "The most interesting trigger [of mystical experience] is sexual lovemaking, interesting because there is virtually no mention of it in the literature on mysticism." He added that research suggested sex was "one of the most frequent triggers of a mystical interlude." He spoke of a mystical experience as a spontaneous, intuitive understanding of the true nature of reality, a sudden insight into "The Way Things Are." We would differ with Greeley slightly: our study suggests that ecstasy may be both a "way" of knowing and the *result* of knowing.

Why has sexual ecstasy been overlooked so long even by

theologians fascinated by this type of experience? People in more sexually repressed times may have thought it immoral to think something as base as intercourse could produce a feeling as elevated as that religious mystics had described. It's also possible that sexual ecstasy was overlooked by mysticism researchers for so long because early studies of mysticism were performed mostly on celibate monks.

Greeley wondered why *everyone* doesn't have such intense sex and concluded it was probably due to the way most people make love. "It is reasonable to presume that much depends on the kind of sex a person has experienced," he observed. "If it is merely a quick and hasty tension release, one could hardly expect anything more to follow. If, on the other hand, an orgasm results from an act of passionate interpersonal love, then it can be reasonably expected that something else might occur. Routine, hasty, furtive, exploitative, anxious sex hardly predisposes a person for anything ... one can, I think, conclude that if there were better sex, one would have to expect ... more mystical experiences." Some 18 percent of the people Greeley studied were having sex so intense they likened it to a mystical experience.

At this point, it's interesting to note that even though peak sex resembles mystical experience, few women in our study specifically equated supersex with religion. They knew that something profound had happened to them, and it certainly had a sacred dimension. The altered state of consciousness experienced during supersex also very much resembles the overwhelming sense of oneness the great Hindu, Christian, and Jewish mystics have reported feeling when communing with God or nature. The women we studied, however, seldom classified these experiences as "mystical": often they simply reported feeling at peace and ineffably at one with themselves, their partners, the universe, and all living things.

Supersex and Other Scientists

At about the same time mysticism researchers like Laski and Greeley were describing men and women enjoying sexual ecstasy, humanistic psychologist Abraham Maslow was defining what he called *peak experiences,* which he also said sometimes occurred during sex. Maslow pointed out that the elements of a peak experience were very similar to the elements of a mystical experience Laski had described. During a peak experience, Maslow noted, it was quite common for a person suddenly to see the entire universe as a unified whole. Maslow spoke of a clarity of mind, a "knowing" that went beyond ordinary daily knowledge, a sense of timelessness, and a feeling of "rightness," that everything was as it should be.

Noting that a peak experience was a more profound feeling than it might sound on paper, Maslow wrote that after even one of these experiences people often came away feeling that "life is worthwhile." He metaphorically likened a peak experience (sexual or otherwise) to "a visit to a personally defined heaven from which the person then returns." But unlike the heaven that many people believe they'll go to after death, Maslow added, the heaven visited during a peak experience "is one which exists all the time all around us, always available to step into for a little while at least."

Maslow also found in his studies that among those people who were reaching the peaks of human potential (those he called "self-actualizers"), marital sex actually got better over the years. He observed, "It is a very common report from these individuals that 'sex is better than it used to be' and 'seems to be improving all the time.' " He concluded that for these people, familiarity with one's partner makes sex not duller, but more interesting. Intriguingly, *supersexual women report the same thing.* Maslow said peak experiences could be brought on by many triggers—from the beauties of nature or a painting to any kind of creative work, including giving birth. But he found the two most common triggers were music and sex.

Another researcher whose theories touched on the experience we call supersex was Stanford University physiologist Julian M. Davidson. In 1980, in an attempt to integrate all the known physiological and psychological data about sexual response available at the time, Dr. Davidson published a chapter in his book *The Psychobiology of Consciousness* in which he observed that human sexual response has many of the same features as an altered state of consciousness. Setting out to establish that human sexual response occurs in the mind as well as the loins, Davidson pointed out that genital arousal alone cannot begin to account for the richness and variety of human sexual experience. He observed what our research has clearly shown: that whether you find sex pleasurable or unpleasurable, satisfying or unsatisfying, exciting or routine depends not just on what's happening to your body, but also on what's going on in your *mind.* As Davidson noted, "the entire body surface is covered with potentially erogenous zones," so no stroke, touch, or nibble is *inherently* "sexy." It's only when our minds interpret a touch or feeling as sexy that we feel turned on. In short, it's not just the body's physiological response, but the interaction of the mind *and* the body that makes a sexual interlude disappointing or joyous.

As a physiologist with a scientific interest in consciousness, Davidson theorized that orgasms and altered states of consciousness often appeared to share many traits. Among them: mood changes, such as euphoria and peacefulness; the capacity to let go; loss of contact with the environment; and the sensations of being "immersed" in the present or "in limbo." Pointing out that the sense of being "lost" during sex resembles that deep state of meditation known as samadhi and that in Oriental tradition (especially Taoism, Buddhism, and Tantric Hinduism) prolonged sexual intercourse has long been used as a way to induce mystical experience, Davidson observed that "the relationship between sex and mysticism is more than trivial."

When Davidson theorized that orgasm should be viewed as an altered state of consciousness, our research suggests, he was certainly on the right track—at least for those attaining the very peaks of sexual pleasure. We cannot draw conclusions about the state of consciousness attained during orgasm because we did not study orgasm directly. But we *do* see supersex as an altered state of consciousness. Clearly, many of the women we studied experience altered states of consciousness not just during orgasm but also before and after orgasmic response. We said it before, but it bears repeating: when these women described sex at its best, many of them mentioned orgasm only as an afterthought.

Hite Found It, Too

Masters and Johnson didn't report people experiencing supersex because they weren't studying sex at its best. They were interested in describing average or typical sexual response patterns. Supersexual women were not the focus of their studies. We found that many supersexual women can fantasize to orgasm without being physically touched at all. One woman told us how she comes to orgasm through fantasy while riding in the backseat of a car or flying cross-country on a plane. Yet in *Human Sexual Response* Masters and Johnson specifically stated that "no woman who can fantasy to advanced plateau stages of sexual tension has been available to [our] investigation."

One sex research pioneer who did discover women reaching supersexual peaks was Shere Hite. When surveying some 3,000 women for her *Hite Report* on female sexuality, published in 1976, she found women who described sex in terms of losing themselves, floating, and feeling their heads separating from their bodies. Hite recognized that these women were experiencing *something* different from an ordinary orgasm. She just didn't know what it was. Grouping these descriptions together in an appendix under the subtitle "Questionable Orgasm Definition Group," Hite wrote: "In a few cases, it was difficult to know with certainty from a woman's answers if she was actually having an orgasm." She then went on to list a number of responses in this category. Among them:

"I feel a sense of physical ecstasy, heat, and I tingle all over, especially my toes."

"I feel lost and floating and not in control of myself and slightly delirious."

"Turning inside out of my body, merging with another or my own mind, falling *up,* about to pass out, then release and relief."

"Feelings vary from gentle floating to complete release from my genitals to my head. It starts in my genitals and streams all over my body. If it's great, it goes up through my head."

"It starts at my toes and sweeps over my body."

"High like floating."

"Orgasms are mind trips with feelings of floating, being separated from all corporal things."

Hite didn't interview these women directly. Her research methodology involved having women fill out written questionnaires. Had she done in-depth interviewing with each subject as we did, she might well have discovered what we now call supersex nearly two decades ago.

In fact, whenever sex researchers have asked people to report how sex feels, they have often come upon a small group describing supersex. In a study published in 1976 in *Archives of Sexual Behavior,* for example, psychologists Ellen Belle Vance, Ph.D., and Nathaniel N. Wagner, Ph.D., asked about 300 University of Washington students to write "a brief statement indicating what an orgasm feels like." From the responses they received, they then randomly chose and published the descriptions submitted by forty-eight students (twenty-four men and twenty-four women). Most of the students described sexual response in terms of a buildup of muscle and genital tension, followed by a physiological release emanating from the genitals. Some typical descriptions falling into this category were:

"Basically it's an enormous buildup of tension, anxiety, [and] strain followed by a period of total oblivion to sensation, then a tremendous expulsion of the buildup with a feeling of wonderfulness and relief."

"Has a buildup of pressure in genitals and involuntary thrusting of hips and twitching of thigh muscles. Also contracting and releasing of the genital muscles. The pressure becomes quite intense—like there is something underneath the skin of the genitals pushing out. Then there is a sudden release of the tension with contraction of genitals with a feeling of release and relaxation."

"A heightened feeling of excitement with severe muscle tension especially through the back and legs, rigid straightening of the entire body for about five seconds, and a strong and general relaxation and very tired relieved feeling."

"A buildup of tension which starts to pulsate very fast, and then there is a sudden release from the tension and desire to sleep."

It appears that most of the students Vance and Wagner studied were describing ordinary, genitally-focused orgasm. A few of their subjects, however, seemed to be describing mind-and-body experiences like those reported by the supersexual women we studied. One would, of course, have to interview each of these students in depth about their most profound sexual moments to determine which ones had gone beyond to attain supersexual ecstasy. But the following student was clearly describing supersex when she or he wrote: "[I] often feel loss of contact with reality. All senses acute. Sight becomes patterns of color, but often very difficult to explain because words were meant to fit in the real world." Students who described "buzzing," "hot-cold tingles," and a complete "blackout" of mental awareness may also have been recalling moments when they experienced supersex.

The Latest Reports

Suddenly in the 1990s, reports of transcendent sexual experiences have appeared in at least half a dozen different books. Most of the descriptions of this sexual phenomenon have come from the New Age literature. In *Sacred Sexuality: Living the Vision of the Erotic Spirit,* for example, California yoga educator Georg Feuerstein, Ph.D., quotes a woman named Deborah who describes one of her best sexual experiences this way:

> Our lovemaking was incredible. Every time we made love, I had an out-of-body trip. It was like moving through space, passing stars and planets until I seemed to be at the center of the cosmos. The universe opened up to me. I saw the Earth being created, saw the early volcanic eruptions and the most angry storms and explosions. It was almost like watching a *Nova* program, except I was *there!*

Another researcher who recently came upon and reported incidents of what we call supersex is writer Dalma Heyn. In her study of married women having affairs, reported in *The Erotic Silence of the American Wife,* Heyn found that once women broke out of their restrictive marriages and had a passionate, illicit romance, some also began enjoying peak sex. One fifty-four-year-old woman named Belinda told Heyn, "I treasure the feelings I have now, how my body gets so filled with colors and feelings." After describing how she hovers on "that edge" between having an orgasm and not having one, she said that as she goes back and forth over the edge and is just about to go over it, "the color . . . starts to shift from the orangey, fiery shades to green and blue like the night sky in December."

Another woman—a forty-six-year-old named Ellie—told Heyn that she sometimes feels as if she's carried

> into a warm sea of blue oil, cozy, Caribbean-colored; and other times, I see rockets with orange and yellow flames. I feel like I'm soaring. There are red rockets in the sky, and it can stop and start like the grand finale of a fireworks display on the Fourth of July in Monaco, a wonderful and continuous spectacle. And I have learned—no, I was taught by my lover—how to keep soaring, what it takes to harness that feeling, to make it like a guided missile—I can now make myself ride that feeling.

Ellie—who is definitely enjoying supersex—gives the credit for her erotic joy to her lover who "taught" her. Her lover may have nurtured the growth in her sexuality, but in the end Ellie taught herself. As many women have learned, the power to enjoy such ecstasy isn't a gift that a woman's partner gives to her; it's a power she carries within.

Another contemporary author, psychologist Margo Anand, describes what she ..as named "High Sex" in *The Art of Sexual Ecstasy* as "a sense of flow . . . comparable to meditation." Of an especially ecstatic moment with her lover, she writes.

Suddenly we both seemed to be floating in an unbounded space filled with warmth and light. The boundaries between our bodies dissolved and, along with them, the distinctions between man and woman.... The experience became timeless.

Anand teaches a path to sexual ecstasy that has emerged through her study of Tantric Sex—an ancient Eastern science of spiritual enlightenment born in India around 5000 B.C. The Hindus believed that the universe was created by the union of the goddess Shakti and the god Shiva. According to this view, Tantra represents the essence of divinity and the central force of all creation. Anand describes how to "contain the energy charge that erotic arousal generates which is normally concentrated in the genitals, and to consciously redirect it through the body using subtle channels that are comparable to the meridians in acupuncture."

So it is clear that we are not claiming to be the first individuals to identify or "discover" sexual ecstasy. It has always existed. References to transcendent sexual experiences can be found in both ancient scripture and more contemporary writings.

What makes this research so unique is the thorough, multidimensional, scientific approach it offers to the understanding of supersex—an elusive, dynamic, transforming phenomenon. Our approach is based upon a cognitive perspective of reality and sexual potential. Supersex is a product of *how we experience* life—our mind-set. Beginning with the discovery of the importance of absorption and centered around hundreds of hours of interviews and analyses of supersexual reports, this research offers an opportunity to expand your own sexual pleasure by sharing in the wisdom supersexual women have revealed to us.

☙ CHAPTER 3 ❧

Women Describe Their Most Passionate Moments

In Ernest Hemingway's *For Whom the Bell Tolls,* the old gypsy woman named Pilar is questioning Maria, a young woman in love with the novel's hero, Robert Jordan. When Maria confesses that when she and Robert made love, she felt the earth move, Pilar replies in mixed Spanish and English that such an experience is very rare, very strange. The two women then continue:

"But it happened, Pilar," Maria said.
"Como que no, hija?" Pilar said. "Why not, daughter? When I was young the earth moved so that you could feel it shift in space and were afraid it would go out from under you. It happened every night."

"You lie," Maria said.

"Yes," Pilar said. "I lie. It never moves more than three times in a lifetime. Did it *really* move?"

"Yes," the girl said. "Truly."

"For you, *Ingles?*" Pilar looked at Robert Jordan. "Don't lie."

"Yes," he said. "Truly."

"Good," said Pilar. "Good. That is something."

"What do you mean about the three times?" Maria asked. "Why do you say that?"

"Three times," said Pilar. "Now you've had one."

"Only three times?"

"For most people, never," Pilar told her. "You are sure it moved?"

"One could have fallen off," Maria said.

In three concise words Hemingway sums up the kind of lovemaking many people dream of all their lives. The earth moved. Those three words say it all. When we asked high absorbers to describe those special moments when the earth moved for them, they all instantly knew what we meant.

We now know from our investigation that Hemingway was mistaken when he wrote that the earth never moves more than three times in a lifetime. Some women had enjoyed these passionate experiences a dozen times, and many reported feeling the earth move every time they make love. But Hemingway was right in saying most people have never found this experience. All of us *could* find it: this potential lies within each of us. It's just that many people have never learned where to look.

Vivid Imagery

During supersex, the minds of the women we studied were filled with intensely vivid imagery—a reflection of their rich inner lives. In addition to fantasizing about sensual body parts or sexual images, these women were reaching the very peaks of sexual ecstasy by becoming lost in a variety of images. Some were lovely, fleeting scenes associated with nature; others were detailed images characterized by intensity, fire, and passion. Two of the women we interviewed actually said they felt the earth move. Darla, a twenty-six-year-old physical education teacher, says that during sex she has a floating sensation and feels tingly all over. But when she finally has what she calls "a whole-body orgasm," she says, "It's like a quivering. My boyfriend describes it as an earthquake. My whole body quivers. I even have these little aftershocks. I do. We'll be lying there after intercourse and I'll be thinking about the sweet time we've just had and I'll get aftershocks."

Another woman, a single, twenty-seven-year-old musician, says, "Lots of times when sex is really intense, I see scenery like clouds, waterfalls, fields, or mountains. I see them in my mind. It's not like I see them when I open my eyes and look around, but I can zoom in on them in my mind. Most of the time, I see a lot of green."

The most often reported images among the supersexual women in our study revolved around liquid, wetness, floating, and ocean waves. "I heard the ocean crashing, and I could smell salt. But we weren't even near the ocean. We were in a cabin in the mountains," recalls Lisa, a twenty-nine-year-old homemaker with a degree in art history. Adelle, twenty-seven, an aerobics instructor married three years to a man with whom she frequently enjoys supersexual peaks, says, "An image just came into my mind which seems like an apt description of how sex feels at its best: it's like liquid fireworks. It's like sparks that come out in liquid form. The sensation starts in my pelvic area and spreads until sometimes I feel it down in my toes. It goes down rather than up [she gestures down and outward], out and down." Angela, thirty-two, says:

I love the ocean. That's my serenity. Sometimes when we're making love, I just go away to a serene place. I think one of the most romantic scenes ever filmed was that one in *From Here to Eternity* where Burt Lancaster and Deborah Kerr are making love on the beach. A lot of times that's where I take my mind. I'm not even in the room anymore. One of these days I'd like to really do that. It's like a fantasy, but it's not like I'm fantasizing that I'm with Robert Redford—not like I'm with somebody else. I'm just at the ocean.

Still another woman says that during supersex, she's just "swimming in the moment, swimming in the sea. I just kind of float there. It's almost like there's an outside force touching my body—like water."

While some supersexual women float, others report seeing fireworks or becoming lost in the stars. Recalling a supersexual experience with her husband of twenty-one years, Susan says, "It was like I was traveling in space." Melanie, twenty-seven, recalls that during one of her best times in bed with a man she dearly loved, "It was . . . how can I describe it? . . . as if I were propelled through space with flashes of color. Like muted stars. Like many, many, many muted colored stars. And afterwards, I said to my lover, 'Wow! That was incredible! What did you do?' He looked kind of puzzled and said, 'I don't know. I didn't do anything different.' [She laughs with delight.] It was great."

Seeing colors during supersex is quite common. Recalling one of her most memorable experiences, which took place one moonlit night in the woods, Wanda, forty-three and a lesbian, says: "I saw colors—a sparkly blue and an intense soft red. Not like a shocking red, but a soft purplish red. It's different every time. But this time the sparks were swirling and had a definite pattern." Helene, forty-three, a piano instructor who loves Emily Dickinson's poetry and Georgia O'Keeffe's paintings, says, "During the really best sex, the colors are like gold and orange. Not red, but sometimes orangey. Also, a lot of gold and white. Bright, hot colors."

Other women don't see colors at all: they simply see white. The soft, peaceful white light Catherine mentioned in the opening chapter was frequently reported. "I always think of white. White comes to mind," says Crystal, thirty-eight. "I've never had fireworks. That never happens for me. But I have *white*. It's very, very vivid, very white." Tina, forty-five, says, "It's not like a flash, but more like a glow of light. More like a pervasive glow. This wonderful flowing white light." Barbara says, "I see white lights. It's just this explosive feeling and white lights. Not stars, not bolts of lightning, but almost like a blank white screen." Jillian, twenty-five, says: "We both just . . . shot out into space. It was like we were out in the universe. We were nothing but light."

Since only a few of the extraordinary women studied make their livings as creative writers, we found this almost universal use of poetic imagery astounding until we recalled that William Wordsworth once defined poetry as "powerful emotion recollected in tranquillity." Simply by describing their most intense moments as accurately as they can, many of these women wind up sounding poetic.

How It Feels . . .

The first step in your own journey to supersexual joy might be to immerse yourself in the stories of the women who've been there. In the extraordinary descriptions that follow, read slowly, and take time to sense what these women may have been feeling as they describe supersexual moments.

Jaclyn, now forty-one, a psychotherapist and self-assured feminist and environmentalist whose fresh-scrubbed, freckled face radiates charm, had the following super-sexual experience at nineteen:

He was the first man who ever got me in touch with my feelings. One time in particular, we were visiting one of his friends' home in Vermont. It was a big, rambling Victorian house with a room over the garage where Mark and I were supposed to stay. We were both in college at the time, and it was right after final exams, so he was just exhausted. And once we got to this room, we lay down on the floor to watch TV and he fell asleep.

I wanted to wake him up gently. So I rolled over, lay partly on top of him, and started rubbing his arms and body very lightly all over. I began to feel almost as if I was in a meditative trance. I could feel his heartbeat and my heartbeat, and I felt our breathing going together. I started moving my hips and body in a way that's hard to describe—very slowly and sensually. It wasn't just a sexual experience. This was *ethereal*. I was there on the floor with him, but I was also on some other plane of existence. And the second he woke up, he was there on that plane with me, and he started moving his hips very slowly and sensuously, too. The feelings I was having weren't even genital-centered. It was like my whole body felt like liquid, but also like fire. My sense of touch was incredibly heightened. Totally spontaneous and relaxed, I felt absolutely no pressure to think about anything or to accomplish anything. There was just this long period of feeling my body flow like liquid fire—almost like floating—on top of his body.

I have no idea how much time passed. It could have been minutes or hours. My guess is that I just floated there for at least half an hour. It was the most incredible sexual experience of my life. And when my orgasm came, it was like no other orgasm I've ever had. You hear all the talk about the G-spot and how it has to be properly stimulated and takes a long time. I don't know. I don't know what kind of orgasm I had—if it was a G-spot orgasm or not. But, I mean, it was out of the top of my head. It just blew my head off. It was unlike any other orgasm has been or ever will be. It was more than physical, this was emotional, spiritual, everything. I was *so* in love with that guy.

A Passionately Married Woman

Margo is a forty-one-year-old novelist who has been married for seventeen years and began experiencing supersex with her husband about ten years ago. Pleasant-faced and attractive, she dresses comfortably yet dramatically, wearing a lot of beautiful fabrics, textures, and colors accented with unusual pieces of jewelry. Though a few pounds overweight, she has no interest in dieting, saying she's come to love her body as it is. Self-employed, she's so busy with her career that she had trouble finding even an hour to be interviewed and asked whether she could send a note describing her most intense sexual moments. Rather than limiting herself to one specific encounter, she describes in the note how she feels almost every time she and her husband make love:

It seems as if everything is working in *harmony*. Neither one of us needs to do anything special. We just let whatever happens happen. What we do unfolds as if I were in a dream and I have no thoughts about doing anything the "right" way or the "best" way. It's as if I'm on automatic pilot and have let go of any conscious control over my actions. I feel my body and my nervous system in synchrony with everything around me. I am unaware of my surroundings or any distractions. Time disappears and we have all the time we need. A moment can be an hour and I have no concept of actual time passing because of my complete involvement in the moment. There is no question of confidence or "how do I look" to my partner, no feelings of worry or fears of failure, no performance goals or feelings of fatigue. Success or orgasm is not an issue and at the same time it's easy to let go and go even deeper into my pleasure. I feel in touch with everything and at one with my actions and my senses. The whole issue of mind and body separation dissolves and I feel both are responding perfectly and naturally to my own inner promptings. At this moment in time, I am acutely aware of colors, sounds, touch, and smells and the feelings of being an unended source of my own pleasure, power, and sexual energy. It is a trance-like state, but I feel totally in touch with everything within and around me, as though all barriers have been pulled away. It is a feeling full of joy, going very deep, and the deeper I go, the higher and higher the sexual intensity.

Supersex and Single Women

Some women like Margo have experienced supersex only in marriage. But for most women, the ability to reach this level of sexual awareness has nothing to do with one's marital status. Stella, a gregarious forty-two-year-old single mother with an infectious laugh and a great sense of humor, has never been married. Yet her descriptions of supersex are among the most vivid of all the women we studied. A leader in both her work and personal life, Stella takes pride in her opinions and attracts people to her because they sense a wisdom she has to offer. She made love for the first time at age fifteen in a swimming pool, and her best sexual moments are still replete with watery images. Here she recounts a recent rendezvous with a college sweetheart she had not seen in seventeen years:

We went to the town where we'd met for the first time. It was one of those romantic things. All the time we'd gone together in college, we were never into romantic symbols like roses or candy. But we *were* always into creating the mood for lovemaking by making sure the setting was very romantic and intimate. This particular time, he had a contractor friend who had just finished building a house. There was no furniture in it, but it was all carpeted, and it was in the middle of a new housing tract where no one else had moved in. I'm one of those people who like for it to be absolutely quiet while we're making love so I can focus on the sounds that are there or aren't there and either add my own sounds or have it be perfectly quiet. It was very dark. Our only light came from a small battery-powered generator we had brought with us. We knew ahead of time we were meeting there to make love, talk, and just commune. And I just remember the *comfort* of knowing that even after seventeen years and even though my body had physically changed, *I* had not changed, my personality was the same. I acted as goofy or as sensual as I would have when I was with him in college, and he was the same way. A lot of little things about him were exactly the same. And yet even though I had all these memories flooding back over me, I wasn't expecting the evening to go in any particular way. If we just continued talking without making love, that would be okay. If he said, "Lie there and let me kiss you toe to head," fine, I'd lie there. My feeling was, "I'm not expecting anything from this evening or this relationship." I think that's what made this evening so perfect: I was just willing to accept whatever might happen.

After talking for a couple of hours and laughing hysterically about old times, we *did* start making love, and it was just as if those seventeen years had never happened. I recognized the knobbiness of his knees [she says this fondly] and the feel of his hair. I recognized the familar smell behind his ears and the salt on his skin; it really was *déjà vu.* At one point I found myself almost floating above us. You know how people always talk about out-of-body experiences? Well, at one point I was on top of him and I looked back and saw myself just standing there *looking* at us. It gave me the eerie feeling for just a moment that somebody else was in the room watching us [she laughs with delight], and I got a little *paranoid.* Then I realized it was just me

standing there, and I think I even laughed. That was unusual for me because I usually make love very quietly. In
fact, he often asks, "Are you breathing?" Sometimes I almost hold my breath for so long he can't tell. He can't even
feel my chest move.

As we made love, all my senses felt keenly alive: the
head-to-toe body contact, the smells, the moisture, the *wetness* of perspiration and body fluids all went along with the
flowing. Everything felt very liquid, I was seeing a lot of
blues, lots of greens, and it was all very enveloping. The
house was near the ocean, so I don't know if I was truly
hearing waves and smelling the salt air, or whether it was
just my imagination. But I could smell salt and hear break-
ers. I just felt immensely calm.

Stella, who sees blues and greens every time she makes
love, speaks of a point during lovemaking—not during orgasm but sometime before it—where "I'm ready to bring
in that extra calmness and my body gets extremely hot on
the outside." Asked what she means by *extra* calmness, she
muses for a while, then replies, "I never thought about it
before. It's just an extra calmness. When my body, mind,
heart, and soul are in sync, I feel absolutely calm. *I* become
the center of what I'm doing, and I totally experience it all."

When Sex Gets Better After Divorce

Nearly every one of the divorced women studied said
sex had gotten better after their marriages broke up. But
these women were already capable—or shortly after their
divorces became capable—of immersing themselves in all
of life's pleasures. If a woman has yet to develop the inner
capacity for pleasure, it's unlikely a divorce alone will
change that.

Elaine, however, is one of the divorcées for whom sex

got better after she left an unhappy marriage. A forty-eight-year-old high school algebra teacher who's about six feet tall, with curly, chestnut-red hair, she has traveled all over the world by herself. She radiates such warmth and spontaneity that it's easy to see why she has so many male and female friends. This experience was with a man she'd been sleeping with about a year and a half and with whom she felt extremely safe:

My children were all upstairs sound asleep. We were downstairs and I'd taken the phone off the hook so we wouldn't be interrupted. It was very quiet and dark. There were no streetlights shining in through the window. The door was locked. I remember his hairy chest, very hairy and hot. My lips on his hairy chest, it felt silky and smelled very, very good. A very delicate scent of soap a few hours old. The heat radiating off his chest felt moist. I ran my fingers down his chest to his belly, where his hair felt thicker, straighter, and softer. Then I remember going down farther into the crisp [pubic] hair and smelling him. Ummmmm, how good—so good, so creamy and fresh and spicy. And tasting him. He tasted like hibiscus with a little bit of slipperiness and that really excited me. I took him in my mouth. He tasted salty, sort of bleachy. Slippery. Hard. I love that smell so much, he tasted so good. I felt him respond and felt the moisture radiate off his body as he began to enjoy it more and more and that really got me excited. I remember thinking, "He loves me so much," and how important that was. He really did, he really *liked* my body. He could amuse himself for hours with his head between my legs, and he loved it. With other men, I sometimes thought they'd kiss me down there because they knew I liked it, not because *they* loved it. But he absolutely loved it. And that made a big difference to me, that he wasn't just pleasing me, that he was doing it for himself, too. We were totally in sync. There was nothing one of us wanted that the other didn't want to do. The flow was perfect. I remember kissing his face and knowing he was smiling in the dark.

We took a couple of hours switching from penetration to oral sex to penetration, back and forth, back and forth, to the point I felt myself transcending this world. I forgot we were in bed. We were tumbling through space together— merged. After one particular orgasm, I remember us clinging to one another, our shoulders touching, and I didn't know which shoulder was his and which shoulder was mine. It was the most profound feeling. All boundaries just melted away. I truly did not know where I stopped and he began. But this wasn't just a physical union, this was a merging of *consciousness*. And all the while that wonderful spicy, almost sweaty smell to his breath.

At the point of orgasm, but it persisted afterward, I had a feeling of tumbling through space. Not a dizzy kind of tumbling. There was no sensation of being in a bed, in a room, or in time. Then, after a while, I remember coming back and realizing there were actually two of us there in the room lying in bed together. I remember kissing a shoulder but still not being sure even then whether it was his shoulder or mine. It was just the most incredible experience of my life. Even though I haven't seen this man for years, I'll always love him because of that experience, just that connection, that bond. It's emblazoned in my mind forever.

Notably, when these women speak of having broken up with a man with whom they've shared such a special connection, the vast majority do not talk with deep regret about "losing" the man or speak of anxiously longing for the day he'll return. Nor do they feel bitter and angry over the fact that he is gone. Instead, these women seem to feel as if sharing supersex just once with a partner somehow brings another dimension to their lives—something that can't be lost. When Elaine says she'll "always love" the man with whom she journeyed to the stars, she's not expressing a need for him to come back into her life—or even a desire to see him again. Rather, she's speaking with the quiet confidence of a woman who knows who she is and doesn't need anyone else to make her feel real or whole. Asked if she'd like to see this particular man again, she replied, "I'd *love* to see him again because he's such a special person, a dear dear friend." But would she sleep with him if they met? "No, probably not. That was another place, another time."

Supersex with the "Wrong" Partner

Supersex can be one strand in the delicate woven fabric of an intricate relationship—but it is *not* the entire relationship. A woman can feel as if she's left her body and flown to the stars with a man and he can still be the wrong partner for life. The supersexual women we studied seem to know this intuitively. Victoria, pregnant with her third child, is a 36-year-old homemaker with well-coiffed ash-blonde hair. She pays careful attention to her makeup and appearance. Well organized and a great cook, she has a home tastefully decorated in soft pastel colors which she finds very calming. She seems to have everything under control, yet she knows to ask for help when she's overextended. Twelve years ago, Victoria was dating a man who, she now recalls, "wasn't good for me in any way." And yet here's how she describes their lovemaking eight years ago on the living room floor:

He was Swedish, about six foot three, bright blue eyes and just exuded sexuality—and he knew it. He had cultivated sex into an art. Sex was always wonderful with him [groan]—always. But this particular night, it was just incredible. We were at his home in Vermont, his mother was asleep down the hall, and there was a soft glowing fire in the fireplace. He and I were lying on the living room floor in front of the fire, just talking, and I mentioned I thought it was sad—and kind of embarrassing really—that I couldn't remember the very first time I'd ever made love. I mean I could remember other times, but I'd forgotten that first time—the one you're supposed to remember forever. We were talking about this, and he'd picked up on the cue. All of a sudden, we were slowly and sensually rubbing against each other and he was talking to me like this was my first time. He was saying all the right words, touching me in all the right ways. As he slowly undressed me, he'd "introduce" me to different erogenous zones of my body, as if I was a virgin who had never experienced sexual pleasure before. He'd say, "These are your breasts and this is how it feels when they're stroked this way. The tip of the breast feels like this when a man lightly runs his tongue over it— like this." And on and on and on. I was getting more and more excited, to the point where I was twenty-two again and I felt as if I'd literally gone back in time. It was almost like someone had hypnotized me. I'm normally quite shy. But if his mother had walked in on us at that moment, I wouldn't even have known she was there. Everything he was doing to me was physical, but it was also emotional. It was like I was riding on a crest. I could just physically feel myself coming out of my body and out of my body and out of my body. I felt my body lift higher and higher until I got to the point where I felt as if I wasn't even in my body anymore. Then all this intense energy inside me drew inward, like a whirlpool. Everything became black, blacker and blacker, until my whole being felt as if it were closing in tighter and tighter into this intense pinpoint of energy. Everything got darker and darker, whirling into this pinpoint of energy, building and building until the pressure got so intense that everything just suddenly Exploded.

Now that she's married to a man she considers her soulmate, Victoria reports feeling this cosmic explosion almost every time she and her husband make love. Still, she says the above experience with the wrong partner was as emotionally and physically charged as it gets.

∞ CHAPTER 4 ∞

Dissecting the Rose

Supersex is a holistic experience of mind, body, emotions, and spirit. If we're to understand this experience fully, we need to examine it in a bit more detail, while keeping in mind that "dissecting the rose" can rob it of its beauty. As you read the following, keep in mind that a woman lost in such a transcendent state does not feel one of these sensations isolated from the others. Rather, she tends to feel a sense of peace *and* timelessness *and* oneness, all together in one overwhelming rush. Like interconnected facets of a diamond or myriad colors dancing through a prism, each part is inextricably linked to the whole. Here are the most commonly reported dimensions of supersexual joy.

A Sense of Timelessness

During supersex there is typically a feeling that one is in a timeless state. Hours seem to fly by in minutes, or in rarer cases, a few seconds can stretch into what seems an eternity. One woman described this feeling as "being lost in the eternal present." Here's how other women report this sensation:

Time just ended. It was a suspension of time. And I'm not just talking about orgasm, I'm talking about the whole feeling.

—Marlene, 47, psychotherapist

Five people could have come in and lined up beside the bed watching, and I wouldn't have even noticed. For me, it literally felt like time had stopped. When I came out of it afterwards, I looked at the clock and thought, "My God, could it really have been over an hour? It felt like five minutes."

—Gwen, 32, editor

I have no idea how much time passed. It could have been minutes or hours. My guess is that I just floated there for at least half an hour.

—Jeanette, 42, interior designer

I don't know how long we made love. I think maybe it was three hours.... We often feel as if we could go on and on.

—Catherine, 39, court stenographer

Everything inside and outside me felt perfectly still, as if the whole universe had stopped. And yet, along with this frozen stillness there was such intense excitement I felt like I'd explode ... a kind of timeless elation.

—Brenda, 36, writer

A Disappearance of Self-Consciousness

We found that during supersex the women in our study let go of self-evaluating "mind-chatter." They weren't constantly asking themselves, "Am I pleasing my partner? Am I doing this right? Do I look okay?" If you've never found that tranquil space inside where self-criticism and self-questioning recede, perhaps these women's words will prompt an exploration of this state of mind.

> We just let whatever happens, happen. What we do unfolds as if I were in a dream and I have no thoughts about doing anything the "right" way or the "best" way.... There is no question of confidence or "how do I look to my partner?", no feelings of worry or fears of failure, no performance goals.
> —*Margo, 41, writer*

> I'm not thinking about how I look or if I'm doing something right for him. I just *am.*
> —*Julia, 34, school administrator*

> It's almost like I'm looking down on us and just feeling good—as if I'm able to shut out all problems and not care where the kids are or that I'm twenty pounds overweight. At these moments, I feel an acceptance of myself.
> —*Beth, 44, homemaker*

> During my best sexual moments, my mind is open—like a hollow tube—and memories and images flow through it freely, with no criticism or pressure.
> —*Sophie, 52, craft store owner*

A Feeling of Being Lost

During sexual ecstasy, a kind of "self-forgetting" also occurs. A woman becomes so immersed in the sensations she's feeling that she may lose awareness of herself, her surroundings, and sometimes even her partner. Paradoxically, by "losing themselves" in the moment, these women find something even more powerful. Joseph Campbell said, "If you realize what the real problem is—losing yourself to some higher end, or to another—you realize that this is the ultimate trial. When we quit thinking primarily about ourselves and our own self-preservation we undergo a truly heroic transformation of consciousness." When women articulate how this heroic transformation of consciousness feels, here's what they say:

> It's like being lost in another dimension. That's often how I feel.... I'm just out there. I don't know how to describe it, but I'm not thinking about anything. I'm just lost in the moment.
>
> —*Danielle, 39, librarian*

> It's a sense of not even knowing where you are because you get totally lost in what you're doing.
>
> —*Lola, 40, dental assistant*

> I was no longer aware of being physically there. It felt like I was kind of floating. I was just aware of our connection and nothing else.
>
> —*Julia, 34, school administrator*

> I had a sense that I was "out there" somewhere. It felt nice to be that carefree. There was no anxiety, no stress, no pressure. There was a freedom in it.
>
> —*Karon, 39, physical therapist*

> My body was physically there, but my mind was gone. A part of me just shot out into the universe.
>
> —*Lydia, 32, office manager*

A Sense of Oneness, Unity, Connectedness

Psychoanalyst Erich Fromm wrote, "The human desire to experience union with others ... is one of the strongest motivators of human behavior.... [We] human beings have lost our original oneness with nature. In order not to feel utterly isolated—which would, in fact, condemn us to insanity—we need to find a new unity: with our fellow beings and with nature." During supersex, at least for a brief time, a woman experiences this sought-after unity. She feels a sense of oneness on many levels—within herself, between herself and her partner, and with the universe.

I feel my body and my nervous system in synchrony with everything around me.... I feel in touch with everything and at one with my actions and my senses. The whole issue of mind and body separation dissolves.... I feel totally in touch with everything within and around me, as though the barriers have been pulled away.

—*Claire, 52, pet shop owner*

We're just so connected. When I'm touching him, I can almost sense what it feels like to be inside his skin being touched by me.

—*Geri, 46, physician*

It was almost like we were one. We were not separate anymore. I wasn't at all concerned with my body. It was just a sense of being one.

—*Lola, 40, dental assistant*

I felt like I was ... transcending some sort of dimension. It was really wild—like the cosmic forces and the universe were opening up in my mind and our souls. At that moment, I have never felt so comfortable and complete.

—*Tobey, 27, housekeeper*

I feel a sense of really merging—not just on a physical level, but a feeling of losing yourself. Where I end and he begins just kind of melt together.

—*Helene, 43, piano teacher*

My feelings weren't at all genitally focused. Our bodies, minds, and spirits were one. We were in total harmony.

—Marcia, 37, carpenter

Relaxed Concentration

Fritz Perls, the father of Gestalt psychology, once said that "trying fails, awareness cures," meaning that the harder we try the more anxious and awkward we become, and that the cure for "trying too hard" can be found in simple awareness. A supersexual woman becomes so focused on sensory pleasures and internal images that she forgets to "try." She simply lets her mind settle into a relaxed, alert state that frees the body to respond naturally.

It's incredible—like a totally relaxed shot of adrenaline. Everything seems just right. It's like nothing could go wrong. I feel like I can do anything.

—Joleen, 32, band instructor

I feel aroused and at peace at the same time. That's the only way I can describe it. My mind is completely alert and yet it's focused only on what we're doing.

—Betty, 48, bicycle shop manager

It's odd because I always thought that to concentrate intensely on anything you had to work to focus your attention. I always believed you had to sort of *beam* your mind directly at what you wanted to concentrate on. But during this particular sexual experience, I felt this intense concentration and alertness throughout my whole body—yet I was amazingly calm and quiet at the same time. It was a feeling unlike any I've ever felt before. It was like my whole body was filled with quiet elation.

—Emma, 28, advertising copywriter

A Sense of "Rightness"

When we asked these women to describe their very best times, they often became perplexingly evasive. They simply would not answer the question. We soon realized why: they consider it meaningless to compare sexual moments as if one were "better" and another "worse." To them, each time they make love is its own special moment.

These women express the conviction that each sexual experience is to be enjoyed purely for what it has to offer: if they achieve an altered state of consciousness, great; if they don't, that's great, too. They view supersex not as a "goal" to achieve, but as a moment to be savored. Jessica, a forty-five-year-old yoga instructor married twenty-one years, puts it this way:

> Those really explosive times where I totally go beyond time and space don't happen every time we make love. But then, they don't have to. I don't go around moping because I'm not always having these experiences. Instead, I treasure every one I have as a real gift. You know, this experience *isn't* a normal, everyday thing. That's what makes it so precious.

Feeling "At Home," Very Safe

Many supersexual women equate the most erotically thrilling moments of their lives with feelings of peace and safety. Only when they feel safe can they let go.

> It's a sense of being psychologically at home.
> —*Naoma, 35, college professor*

> The rest of the world doesn't exist and it's like I'm in a sort of *cocoon* for a brief window of time.
> —*Jackie, 44, realtor*

I had a very strong feeling everything was okay—that nothing could go wrong. [This from a woman who often worries that things will go wrong.]

—Bea, 33, homemaker and mother of two

A Sense of "Knowing"

"The best things can't be told because they transcend thought," Joseph Campbell said. That's certainly true of supersex. Women frequently mention the ineffable quality of these experiences. "I can't describe it," they'll say. During supersex, a woman often senses that she and her partner are communicating at a level of meaning so deep it's beyond words. There's often a sense that a woman and her partner are in such perfect rhythm that each intuitively "knows" what the other is thinking. There's also a sense that the woman is in touch with some deeper level of reality, that for at least a few moments she understands life more completely.

A lot of times we sort of have to negotiate when we'll make love: He'll want to do it, and I'll be too tired, or I'll be turned on and *he'll* have a headache. Yet this particular night, we were both tired and yet suddenly we just had this incredible passion. It was very spontaneous, sudden, passionate, and intense. We just looked at each other and we knew we wanted to make love, and we knew we were both feeling a very intense passion. I looked at him, he looked at me, and we *knew.*

—Ingrid, 30, girls' basketball coach

You know, in sign language, we say *aha,* which means "I understand." It means, "I get it." And for a moment, you get it—you understand reality—in a way you didn't before. Things have become clearer.

—Leila, 45, artist

During these peak moments, we don't have to say a thing. He just seems to "know" what will build my excitement. It's a kind of communication beyond words.

—Pauline, 38, attorney

Everything we did was just right for both of us. It wasn't like one of us wanted to do one thing and the other didn't.

—Ina, 50, secretary

One of the most fascinating stories of a woman's "just knowing" the seemingly unknowable was told to us by Leila, forty-five, who has been deaf from birth:

I was with a man named Jason in New York. And I knew at the very moment it happened that I was pregnant. Before we had an orgasm, I knew I was pregnant, and he knew it, too. It was like this connection with each other. Without words, we knew. This went way past a physical sensation ... it was very, very spiritual. My mind and body reacted differently than they ever had before during sex. It was like I was floating, in my mind. I can't really describe it. But God was with me. I was so far away, my mind was a blank, but at that moment—right before we climaxed—I knew I was pregnant. I felt my body suddenly change. I just looked at him and he looked at me, and we both knew. In the middle of the night I found myself waking up and not knowing what time it was. He was still inside me and we were just frozen like that in time. In the morning, he said he would be a father and I would be a mother. And we both knew it was true.

Although some supersexual couples may experience an effortless sense of "knowing," we're not suggesting that this is the way they *always* communicate, or that clear verbal communication—including exchange of sexual preferences, feelings, or concerns—is somehow unnecessary. They are not just "mind readers." On the contrary, the most satisfying sexual connections usually reflect a level of communication and commitment that is a product of *both* partners' investment in their relationship. These are couples who have chosen to make a special place for each other and for their intimacy. Even in the midst of busy schedules, they tell us they have made certain to give sexuality a "high priority" in their lives. Instead of squeezing their lovemaking into a space between emptying the dishwasher and paying the bills, they try to set aside special time for themselves as a couple. What they have discovered is that the more they make time to touch and to share feelings or personal thoughts, the more often these moments of "just knowing" emerge.

CHAPTER 5

Supersex, Peak Performance, and Flow

It is difficult to name or to exactly define experiences as in-effable as those these women have described, because of the baffling sense that to name or define it is also to limit or diminish the phenomenon. As semanticist Alfred Korzybski has pointed out, things are not what we *say* they are: language merely represents our thoughts. Just as you cannot really *know* what water is until you drink it or *know* sweetness until you taste it, you can only know supersex by experiencing it.

And yet, if we're to make this experience ours—especially if we've never tasted it before—it helps to give it a name. Clearly, what the women we studied described is *more* than an intense orgasm or multiple orgasms. So what is it? Are the perceptions these women have during supersex illusions? Have their five senses been somehow distorted by passion? Are they so absorbed in the moment that they're cut off from reality? And if so, why do they so often report feeling a *heightened* awareness—a sense that they suddenly understand life more completely?

Over the past fifty years, psychologists have given such experiences various names. The most familiar of these are *peak performance, flow,* and *peak experience.* The state of consciousness these three experiences share is much like the state of mind the women we studied reported. But even though these three experiences are related to supersex, they also differ in some key ways. Let's examine these concepts more closely.

Peak Performance

In many ways, the sensations women report during supersex—the quiet mind, letting go, and sense of timelessness—sound a lot like the sensations Olympic athletes, composers, and others report when performing at their very best.

In *The Silent Pulse,* George Leonard tells the story of Richard, who had made it to a pre-Olympic track meet in Mexico City. "It was a tremendous strain," Richard recalled. "Here we were in a strange city, in a strange climate, eating strange food. The day of the finals I ran *six* races—quarterfinals and semi-finals." At the time of the seventh race—when he was so exhausted he had nothing left to give—he experienced a sudden shift of consciousness. "There was a strange sense of completion," Richard told Leonard. "It was as if I was in the exact center of time, there was just as much in front of me as in back of me. It's hard to explain. All potential in front of me was equal to all time in back of me, and I was balanced in the center. Having given in, I didn't have to relate to winning or representing my country. I was just *there.* The starter's gun went off and I watched myself run the race, running in the center of time. Everything was so precious—my breath, the sky, my relationships, my life." When he won the race, Richard realized it wasn't the winning that mattered. What mattered was having experienced this remarkable moment.

Elaine likens a peak sexual experience to the feeling she gets when she's running and goes through "the runner's wall." She explains, "It's like you could go on forever. You feel this intense sense of heightened awareness—a tremendous power." Natalie, who swims about a half mile every morning, says the quiet state of mind she reaches when making love resembles the feeling she often has while swimming laps. "When I first dive in the pool, all my muscles feel coiled and tense and it's an effort to move through the water," she says. "But after about the sixteenth twenty-five-meter lap, my whole body begins to feel very loose and free, and the water begins to feel 'soft.' That's the only way I can describe it—it feels almost like a down pillow. Slicing through the soft water becomes so effortless it's almost like I'm not even swimming with my body anymore: it's like I'm swimming with my *mind*. And yet at the same time, my mind is crystal clear." Natalie adds, "Peak sex differs from swimming in that when I'm making love I'm a lot more physically and emotionally excited and I become so lost in the moment I don't even know where I am. But that clarity of mind is the same."

Yet even though peak performance resembles supersex in many ways, there are shades of difference.

First, during peak performance, people usually report being acutely aware of their surroundings. When jogging through the park, for example, a runner may find that the rocks, sky, trees, and path beneath her feet all seem more clearly "real," colors are more vivid, and lines seem sharper. During supersex, however, women are so focused on the passionate feelings *inside* that their surroundings usually just disappear. As Ingrid, the thirty-year-old girls' basketball coach, recalls: "One minute we were on the floor and the next minute we were on the bed. And when I was on the hardwood floor, you would think it would be so *hard*. But it wasn't, because I was not even focused on the fact I was on the floor. I kept my eyes open because I really like looking at him, I like the connection. I was just totally aware of him. I was not aware of the bed or the color of the sheets or even what end of the bed we were on. It was as if everything had just melted away, and I wasn't even aware of my surroundings."

Second, peak performers tend to feel *more* self-aware, whereas supersexual women usually have a transitory sense of *losing* themselves. A peak performer might say, "I felt incredibly powerful—as if I could do anything," whereas a supersexual woman would more likely recall, "I wasn't anywhere anymore. I was just *gone.*" Rather than feeling more self-aware during supersex, you may feel as if you're *transcending* yourself—as if you're connected to the entire universe.

Third, according to University of West Florida psychologist Gayle Privette, who has been investigating different types of peak experiences for more than twenty years, peak performance is usually—although not always—a solitary pursuit. Whereas supersexual women enjoy masturbation—and a few even reported that when masturbating they felt a "cosmic connection"—the vast majority of these women find sex more intense with a partner. Felicia, forty-seven, explains this best when she says, "For me, it's the interplay [that makes sex most intense]. For me, it is that feeling of I-Thou, so there has to be a Thou."

The Connection to Flow

Another experience that closely resembles supersex is that psychological state which University of Chicago psychologist Mihalyi Csikszentmihalyi calls "flow." He defines flow as "the holistic sensation that people feel when they act with total involvement." The "flow" state is characterized by several key dimensions: intense involvement; deep concentration; clarity of feedback; and an altered sense of time. Hours can seem like minutes or minutes like hours.

Flow involves anything you do just because it feels good and you enjoy it: working, playing chess, rock climbing, reading, you name it. Flow ranges along a scale of complexity—from moments of "microflow," which can involve a pleasure as simple as chewing a stick of your favorite gum, to episodes of "deep flow," which represent the highest levels of complexity a human being can achieve. One example of deep flow might be that state of ecstasy the great mystics are reported to achieve when they feel a oneness with God. After studying people all over the world, Dr. Csikszentmihalyi has concluded that flow is the very secret of happiness. The more time we spend in flow, he explains, the more happy, meaningful, and complete our lives will be.

People in flow often sound remarkably like women describing supersex. Some examples from Csikszentmihalyi's research: "Perhaps the best part of it is that I feel I could go on doing it until I am completely exhausted" (this said by a student about playing soccer and volleyball); "I felt we were one, that we were united. She was a creature to be loved" (said by a blind woman caring for a gravely ill friend); and "You cannot judge in terms of some final goal; it is the moment-by-moment rightness that makes you feel good" (said by a Turin art student about drawing).

A key quality which flow shares with both supersex and peak performance is absorption—a sense of being so totally involved in what you're doing that you lose all sense of your surroundings. As one chess player told Csikszentmihalyi, "The concentration is like breathing—you never think of it. The roof could fall in and, if it missed you, you would be unaware of it."

Csikszentmihalyi calls such experiences *flow* because people so often use this word when recalling these moments. And indeed, when describing peak sex, women often use this term, too.

> There was just this long period of feeling my body flow like liquid fire—almost like floating—on top of his body.

> There was nothing one of us wanted that the other didn't want to do. The flow was perfect.

> Memories and images flow through [my mind] freely, with no criticism or pressure.

People in flow frequently mention that "loss of self" supersexual women describe. According to Csikszentmihalyi, one of the crucial elements of flow is that "concern for the self disappears, yet paradoxically the sense of self emerges stronger after the flow is over." Recalling the flow experience he had while scaling a mountain, for example, one rock climber said, "You are so involved in what you are doing you aren't thinking of yourself as separate from the immediate activity. . . . You don't see yourself as separate from what you are doing." Conductor Leonard Bernstein was also talking about being in flow when he said, "The only way I have of knowing I've done a really remarkable performance is when I lose my ego completely and become the composer. I have the feeling that I'm creating the piece, writing the piece on stage, just click, click, making it up as I go, along with those hundred people who are also making it up with me." His perceptions sound similar to those of one young supersexual woman who told us, "Often when I'm dancing, I'm not just listening to the music, I'm *acting* the music. It's like I'm the person singing the song and the musicians playing the instruments. I *am* the music."

Supersexual experience seems to be a form of "deep flow," but again this psychological concept doesn't fully encompass supersexual bliss. According to Csikszentimihalyi, two key requirements of flow are that a person "set goals" and "seek new challenges"—ideas that could easily block supersexual ecstasy entirely by increasing performance anxiety. During supersex, there are no goals nor challenges: there is only the joy of being.

Peak Experience: The Concept That Comes Closest

Of all the names given to those times when humans function at their very best, Abraham Maslow's idea of a peak experience comes closest to the feelings supersexual women describe.

One key aspect of peak experience is, again, absorption—the ability to block out all distractions and become totally focused on the moment. During a peak experience, according to Maslow, a person becomes so completely absorbed that she feels outside time and space. Setting aside critical judgment, she becomes fully accepting and loving: everything feels perfect, complete, exactly as it should be. There is also such a sense of wonder and awe that all fear, anxiety, and self-consciousness just slip away. Intense aliveness, lack of straining, and a feeling of being totally open and honest are all dimensions of any peak experience. People who have had peak experiences frequently speak of transcending themselves and feeling profound ecstasy—a sense that life has a deeper meaning than we often notice in our daily lives. Quite often, Maslow also noted, "the entire universe is perceived as an integrated and unified whole."

One of the youngest of the supersexual women we interviewed—an eighteen-year-old English literature major named Hillary—recalls having this peak experience one morning while walking across her college campus:

I was just strolling across the quad on my way to class. Hundreds of other students were also walking around. They weren't noticing me or anything. And I just got this sudden revelation that everyone's heart was beating. You know how if you think about some part of your body—your hand, for example—you can feel it more because you're thinking about it more? Well, it was like we were all focusing on our hearts and I suddenly realized they were all beating together. But it was more than that. It was like there was this invisible thread connecting all of our hearts together. And it wasn't just those people in the quad, it was everybody in the whole world. You know how sometimes you have a feeling but you're not quite sure whether it's real or not? Well, this was *real*. I knew it was real. I got a kind of rush from it.

At times a peak experience can be so transforming the person is never quite the same again. Naoma, who teaches journalism in a small college, says the following peak experience was like a "wake-up call" that has given her life richer meaning:

> I was forty-four, and for the past couple of years I'd been on a real search for meaning in my life. All the old answers no longer seemed to fit, but I didn't have any new ones. I'd been reading Martin Buber, Schopenhauer, Carl Jung, and a lot of other writers. I'd also become absolutely fascinated with the new physics as it's described in *The Tao of Physics* and *The Dancing Wu Li Masters.* One famous physicist said that the more he studies the universe the less it looks like a giant machine and the more it begins to look like a giant brain. Some physicists believe that at the very smallest, subatomic levels of reality, matter is dancing *in and out* of existence. Modern physics has become almost mystical.
>
> Anyway, I was sitting in my backyard one afternoon, gazing at the sky, thinking about all this and wondering what it might mean when I suddenly *felt* how interconnected the whole universe was. This was one of those experiences, as they say in the *Upanishads,* from which "words turn back." There are no words to fully describe it. But it was like I felt the whole universe dancing around me. And God was part of it, and I was part of it, and so was everyone and everything else. At that moment I realized that every second we're alive—even during all those times we're worried and upset and thinking we've made a mess of our lives— everything's really okay because we're all involved in this incredible cosmic dance. And I felt a kind of happiness I'd never felt before: it was ecstatic joy coupled with a deep inner peace. It's hard to explain. But for a long time after that I no longer felt I had to *search* for the meaning because I had *experienced* the meaning. Do you understand what I'm saying? It was unbelievably awe-inspiring.

Since this experience, Naoma says, "I feel a lot more centered and content. Sure, I still have times in my life— especially when I'm rushing to finish a project—that I'm so anxious my stomach churns. But there are many days now when I can just take a deep breath and let it all go. I've learned that most of the problems we tie ourselves up in knots over aren't nearly as important as we'd like to believe."

Of all the psychological concepts developed to describe such joyous times in one's life, peak experience is the one that comes closest to what the women we studied experienced sexually. Yet somehow, just classifying these moments as "peak sex" seems insufficient. Reading descriptions like Hillary's and Naoma's, one senses the possibility of an even greater mystery.

Supersex as the Ultimate Connection

The supersexual women we studied frequently used such phrases as "all boundaries melted away," "our hearts beat in unison," and "I felt cosmic forces and the universe opening up in my mind and our souls." Can we dismiss such descriptions as delusions or mere metaphor? Perhaps, but at the risk of judging prematurely. Evidence from a variety of scientific sources suggests that these self-reports may be more than metaphors.

When Jaclyn says she felt her lover's heart beating "at one" with her own, she may have been sensing a kind of synchrony that sometimes occurs when two or more people are moving rhythmically together. Dr. Paul Byers, a researcher in non-verbal communications at Columbia University, reports that during rhythmic activities such as rowing, singing, and marching, people's breathing will sometimes synchronize. Most women recall instances, often from their college days, when a number of women living in close quarters got their periods at the same time because their menstrual cycles had synchronized. George Leonard, past president of the Association for Humanistic

Psychology, has written: "When two individual muscle cells from the heart are observed under a microscope, each pulses with its own separate rhythm. Yet when they are moved closer, they begin to pulse together, perfectly synchronized." Byers notes it has also been observed that when a psychotherapist and patient are "in sync," their hearts beat in unison.

The same kind of synchronization—or what some scientists call *entrainment*—will occur between two pendulum clocks hanging side by side on a wall. Imagine you've set the two clocks at approximately the same time so that their pendulums are swinging in almost the same arc. If you leave the clocks on the wall for a few days, then come back, you'll discover that the pendulums are swinging in exactly the same arc. This phenomenon, first observed in 1665 by Dutch scientist Christiaan Huygens, is in fact universal. When two or more oscillators are close to each other and pulsing in almost the same rhythm, they'll tend to "lock in" until they're pulsing in exactly the same rhythm. Why? Because nature tends to move toward a state requiring the least energy to maintain, and it takes less energy to pulse together than in opposition.

Given these explorations, we surmise that some of these supersexual women and their lovers perhaps *have* felt their hearts beating as one.

Some supersexual women reported feeling what one called "a sense of wholeness, as if everything in the universe is connected and I'm part of it all." We could dismiss this as metaphor. But when we asked these women whether they were using metaphors, they told us they weren't. "I'm not trying to be poetic," Naoma said of the experience described earlier in this chapter. "I'm trying to tell you as clearly as I can how I felt. I really *did* feel a connectedness with the universe and all living things and I *knew* it was true. It wasn't like later I said, 'Wow, what a feeling—I wonder if that really happened?' I *knew* it was true. No one could ever convince me otherwise. For that brief moment of time, I *knew* the essence of the universe was wholeness, rhythm, and connectedness, and I'll never forget it. I'll always carry the joy and peace of that moment inside me."

When some of these women report feeling a sense of "wholeness with the universe" and "connectedness" with all living things, their ideas are remarkably close to ones which many scientists have entertained. When Albert Einstein was alive, for example, he was considered by many "the smartest man in the world," so he often got letters asking him questions. One came from a rabbi who explained that he had tried every way he could think of to comfort his nineteen-year-old daughter after the death of her younger sister, but the girl was inconsolable. In a letter to the rabbi, Einstein wrote:

> A human being is part of the whole, called by us "Universe".... He experiences himself, his thoughts and feelings as something separate from the rest—a kind of prison for us, restricting us to our personal desires and to affection for a few persons nearest to us. Our task must be to free ourselves from this prison by widening our circle of compassion to embrace all living things and the whole nature in its beauty. Nobody is able to achieve this completely, but striving for such an achievement is in itself a part of the liberation and a foundation for inner security.

Citing this letter in his book *Full Catastrophe Living,* Dr. Jon Kabat-Zinn, founder and director of the stress reduction clinic at the University of Massachusetts Medical Center, wrote: "[In his reply, Einstein] is not belittling the suffering we experience at such a loss. But he is saying that our overwhelming preoccupation with our own separate lives ignores another, more fundamental level of reality. . . . Einstein is reminding us to see wholeness as more fundamental than separateness." Of course, Kabat-Zinn observed, we *are* separate in that we have separate bodies and live unique lives; but "Einstein is reminding us that when we neglect the perspective of wholeness and connectedness, we only see one side of being alive."

ᗌ CHAPTER 6 ᗡ

Supersex and Beyond: Bringing Passion to All Experience

There is a pertinent saying in one of the Upanishads: *"When before the beauty of a sunset or of
a mountain you pause and exclaim, Aha!, you
are participating in divinity." Such a moment
of participation involves a realization of the
wonder and sheer beauty of existence.*

—Joseph Campbell

Supersexual women frequently report peak experiences
not only while making love but also at nonsexual times in
their lives. They seem to be connecting more deeply not
just with their lovers, but with all of life.

Twenty-eight-year-old Trisha, a writer who worked for
six months as a reporter on a Venezuelan newspaper, told
us how her perceptions during supersex differ from those
during other peak experiences.

The first experience Trisha describes occurred one
summer night when she was sleeping alone under the
stars beside a river in the Sierra Nevada:

> Suddenly, I heard a loud crash in the woods. I peered out
> into the darkness and, among all these boulders beside the
> river, I saw one that looked particularly large and dark.
> Then it moved, and I saw the silhouette of a bear about
> twenty feet from me. It was huge. I was looking at its shoul-
> der and thinking, "It's so beautiful." I was so mesmerized

by the way this bear moved, I totally forgot about the danger I was in. I was frozen in time. Then I realized I had to get away from there fast because he was headed my way. But for a few seconds that seemed to stretch into hours I forgot—because it was so beautiful—that I was about to be trampled by a six-hundred-pound bear.

A second experience took place when Trisha was sixteen and swimming alone one night in the dark:

I was floating on my back and I started spinning in the water, going round and round. The phosphorescence was lighting up the plankton in the water and the stars were shining brilliantly overhead. I thought I was face down in the water looking at the plankton, so I breathed out. But I was actually face up looking at the stars. All of a sudden, my lungs filled with air and I just felt propelled up in space. I was only sixteen at the time, but I'll always remember it. I was astounded.

Later, Trisha describes the distinctions she draws between supersex and other peak moments:

To me, [supersexual ecstasy] is akin to having an out-of-body experience—that is, completely forgetting one's surroundings, perhaps even who one is, and feeling that your soul belongs to all that was and will be. A connection with eternity, I suppose. Sexual peaking can be achieved for me only if I feel good about myself and who I am with. During such an experience, I have felt propelled out into the universe—I'm not sure *where,* really (a place in my mind, I suppose)—with stars, cosmic matter, lights with colors rushing and exploding everywhere. It's almost like a river of exploding colored lights rushing through my brain. That's what I saw inside my head during the peak sexual experience. During other peak experiences—other than sexual—these cosmic lights did not occur. But I had the experience of forgetting I was on the physical plane, "unencumbered" by my body. I think this is the prelude to peak experiences, and each one plays itself out differently according to the circumstances surrounding it. The rushing lights occurred during sex. Temporarily forgetting to remove my body from an approaching bear or feeling propelled into the universe by floating on my back and looking at the stars were all peak experiences to me, and all began with forgetting that I exist on the material plane. None of these experiences were premeditated. I don't think that's possible for me at this point. Maybe one day I'll be able to "fly about" just sitting at the kitchen table, but not now.

Moments of extreme danger—that is, feeling "I might die" seem in and of themselves to cause me to forget the physical plane. I recall a particularly dangerous situation from which I removed myself and then, without hesitation, I walked back into it. I was reporting on the riots in Caracas [in 1989] and the streets were filled with tear gas, bullets, flying rocks and bottles, burning buses. I felt at that point a pressing need to leave the scene. It was mayhem because everyone else was feeling the same need. There was a woman walking in the direction of the most serious conflict. I had supposed she lived in a building nearby. But she stopped me and said, "Someone told me the metro was over there." In fact, it was through the underpass (in the area of conflict). The place was also filled with military police. At first, not wishing to return that way, I pointed out the direction. And then I noticed a tiny infant tucked under her shirt. She also had a large sack. For some reason, to this day I don't know why, I said, "Perhaps someone could help." Then I took the sack and walked her to the metro. There was no hesitation, no fear. I suppose maybe it was just my needing to see the infant to safety that drove me to do it, because after they went in I turned around and thought, "Oh, God! How do I get out of here?"—as if I had no idea how I had arrived back in the area of conflict! For that three-block walk I had forgotten my existence on the physical plane and was shocked back into it once I "came to my senses," as it were. I regard this as a peak experience because it fits my criterion of forgetting that my body houses my spirit. This was not an enjoyable peak experience. In fact, the only thing that remains utterly clear is wondering why I was at the metro station in the first place. So it occurs to me that peak experiences can occur anytime. They don't have to be gleaned from pursuits of enjoyment. And further- more, I don't seem to have control over *when* they happen. Maybe lack of premeditation and control are essential fac- tors of peak experience. For me, peak experiences happen when I forget who and where I am. I seem to come away from them wondering, "Just *where* did I go? Was that me?"

The women we studied often likened supersex to other profound moments they'd experienced. But, like Trisha, a twenty-seven-year-old attorney named Marcie also draws a clear distinction between the two feelings. During supersex, she says, "I see a white light—not a flash, but more like a pervasive glow of light." Then she adds, "I re- member that same sort of feeling, only without the physi- cal sensation, when I was meditating in a yoga class I'm taking. It was just like this peaceful kind of light—flowing, whitish, yellowish light. I remember lying on the floor and it very much felt like the light was coming out of the cen- ter of me. It was incredible. I felt wonderful afterwards."

Other women described having similar feelings when they're alone outdoors. At age fourteen, Samantha was sexually molested by an uncle. Traumatized and feeling unlovable, she slept with twenty-two men during her teens and her early twenties. Now, at age twenty-four, she says one supersexual encounter coupled with experiences like the following have helped her realize that life—even when it's painful—has a deeper purpose and meaning.

I was sitting on the beach with my dog, watching the surfers play and the sunset. Normally my dog is just real feisty, always running and barking. But this particular day we were both just staring into the water. The next thing I knew it was half an hour later, and both of us were still sitting there. There was just this incredible sense of calm and peace. I felt a part of something bigger. It gave me the chills to think how minute I was compared to the vastness of nature. And yet I felt like I was a part of it all.

Samantha says, "I carry that peace I felt at the beach with me all the time now because I feel good about myself. It's been over two years now that I've felt this way. I've learned that I could not be the woman I am today if it weren't for everything—good and bad—that has ever happened to me. Nothing that happened when I was a child can hurt me anymore because I am lovable, I am a good person, and I should never have felt that I wasn't."

Elaine had a similar experience. She recalls, "After reading *Fear of Flying* by Erica Jong, I remember almost *awakening* to my sensuality. Like with babies, I remember always enjoying their smell. But when I started this awakening, I would just *inhale* the smell of their hair and just resonate with that smell. So this awakening didn't just take place in sex, it involved other parts of my life." She says supersexual experiences along with experiences like the one that follows "make me appreciate and value life more."

I have a favorite beach down on Long Island called Meadowbrook. It's a bird sanctuary where there are no concession stands. And I remember, after this awakening began, walking down that beach and becoming euphoric, similar to the euphoria of sexual arousal. The sky was brilliant blue, the waves were crashing, the sand underfoot was cool and crunchy, and the breeze was soft with that salty smell. There was nothing harsh on the skin. There were a few people around, a few children playing in the water. But there were no bikers, no loud radios playing. It was a very safe place—nothing threatening. I just felt so peaceful and alone. All of the troubles, heartache, and hardness of life was, for twenty-five minutes maybe, truly gone.

Sandra, a thirty-three-year-old electrical engineer working for a Fortune 500 manufacturing company, describes the following incident while driving home one evening:

It was just about dusk and I remember feeling very relaxed. Listening to my radio as I drove along a familiar road canopied with lovely old trees—oaks, elms, maples—I suddenly began to feel a "tingling" that I can only describe as a mild electrical shock (maybe I describe things that way because I'm an electrical engineer). [she laughs] The sensation came on swiftly and seemed to be radiating from my belly. It felt warm, comforting, and inviting—almost *spiritual.* I decided to turn off the radio to make the moment more peaceful, slowed my car, and concentrated on this strangely pleasant feeling. Just then I began to have the sensation of *expansion*—I really can't describe it in any other way—as if I were becoming physically bigger. I had no sense of alarm; it felt very natural. As I continued to "grow," I had the spontaneous sense that I could "connect" with the trees above me. I briefly raised my hands from the steering wheel and tried to "touch" them as I passed beneath. I had never had such a feeling before. It was fantastic! It was as if I could actually feel life's energy at my fingertips! Then, as suddenly as the experience had started, it ended. I seemed to be jerked back to the present by the need to steer the car.

In that one moment, Sandra discovered that there was a spiritual connection beyond what she had originally thought to be possible, a connection with the universe that was within her. She has not experienced supersex yet (she's looking for a partner), but she's a woman who has discovered an unbounded capacity to enjoy life.

During such intense moments, women often seem to be standing in what mystic Martin Buber called an "I-Thou" relation to the world and those around them. You'll recall

Felicia's comment that during sex she has to have "that feeling of I-Thou."

Essentially, Buber says we can relate to the world and each other in one of two ways: *I-It* or *I-Thou*. When we're in an *I-It* relationship, we want to control, possess, use, own, or "have" whatever we're relating to. We usually have an *I-It* relationship, for example, with our possessions, such as money or a new car. But because this is the dominant way of addressing life in our culture, it's very easy to carry this *I-It* stance over to everything in our lives: to make friends with people who can further our careers, to try to own and control our children, to "possess" happiness in an attempt to "have" a successful life. When addressing life in an I-It mode, Buber says, one takes in only the fragments of an experience. When seeing a sequoia tree as an It, for example, we might marvel at how tall it stands, how rough and red its bark looks, or how ancient it appears: we see separate characteristics of the tree. But we don't truly *see* the essence of the whole tree.

Our language reveals how much of our lives most of us spend in this *I-It* mode: we talk about our need to have friends, have a relationship, have fun, have orgasms. Yet beneath our desires to have, our language also reveals that on some level we know we could be experiencing a deeper, more meaningful relation with life: underneath it all, we understand we can only *be* happy.

I-Thou is the realm not of having, but of being. When you're relating to the world in an *I-Thou* mode, you have no interest in trying to control, use, own, or change. You simply stand in reverence. You directly experience the world. You simply *are*. We've all had moments like this in our lives when we've seen an exquisite painting, a newborn baby's face, or some other experience, and our minds become absolutely still as we say, "Ah!" In such *I-Thou* moments, Buber says, we no longer see the separate qualities of the tree, such as the bark, the branches, and the green leaves against the blue sky: we simply stand in relation to the whole tree. The tree reaches out and "grabs" us, if you will—seizes our attention—and we understand the unique essence of that one particular tree. Leila, who told us about the night she "just knew" she was pregnant, recently had an experience with a tree which sounds much like the *I-Thou* relationship Buber refers to:

Last October, I went to Vermont. I'm from California, and it was the first time I'd ever seen autumn foliage. I remember one Saturday morning in a motel, I opened a window, put up the shade, and there was this one yellow tree. It was very bright yellow. Just one. Nothing else was around—just that one tree. As I sat on the corner of the bed, watching that tree, I began smoking. I had an ashtray on the windowsill. And I was just looking, letting myself go into the tree. It was beautiful. I don't know how long I sat there, just staring at that tree, but when I woke up and came out of the tree, I had a pile of cigarettes up to here. [She indicates the ashtray was full.] I know from measuring the time by the number of cigarettes I smoked, it must have been hours and hours and hours. It was sort of like that movie *The Ten Commandments,* where Moses talks to the burning bush. It was such a bright yellow. The day was overcast, and I was just gone.

Listening to Sandra's and Leila's experiences, we recalled yet another bit of wisdom from Joseph Campbell: "The Indians addressed all of life as a 'thou' (an object of reverence)—the trees, the stones, everything. You can address anything as a 'thou,' and if you do it, you can feel the change in your own psychology. The [self] that sees a 'thou' is not the same [self] that sees an 'it.' " The self that sees an "it" is the limiting self, which stands separate from others. The self that sees a "thou" is the true self, which feels the connection of all living things.

How does all this relate to going beyond conventional boundaries and achieving your full sexual potential? Once you sense how it feels to relate in an *I-Thou* mode in any area of your life, you can use this inner understanding to enrich and deepen your appreciation for all of life. And that includes the way you relate sexually to another human being.

∽ CHAPTER 7 ∽

What's the Partner's Role?

Joy in sex is experienced only when physical intimacy is at the same time the intimacy of loving.

—Erich Fromm

You might think that because sex gives these women such exquisite pleasure, they want to make love nonstop with any partner they can find. But in fact, supersexual women tend to be sexually selective. A few have slept with a dozen or more people, but the vast majority, even when they're single, are serially monogamous and quite discriminating about the people with whom they make love.

Serena, who has had sexual relationships with both women and men, says, "In my sex life, I don't run around. You know, some women use themselves and abuse sexual feelings. I can't do that. I make a commitment to one person, and I can't accept anyone else. My sexuality is too *special* for me to enjoy casual sex."

Many of these women feel they have a kind of internal radar that sounds an alarm when it comes to selecting a partner. Felicia laughs as she recalls, "I had one fellow following me around saying he wanted me to be his kundalini partner, and I turned him down flat. He had the words, but he didn't have the feeling for me, and I wasn't interested in helping somebody else 'transcend.' I wanted something for me."

To reach that deep state of focused relaxed concentration described in supersexual moments, a woman needs to suspend critical judgments ("Will I have an orgasm? Do I look okay? Am I pleasing my partner in the right way?"), stop *striving* to make sex sensational, and open herself to whatever the moment might bring. Rather than trying to *control* lovemaking, she needs to let the *experience show her the way. The experience of supersex is inside all of us, if we can ask our critical selves to retreat.*

What does the partner have to do with all of this? A woman's partner facilitates her ability to "let go" by providing a safe, trusting setting. In order to open deeply to passion, most women in our sample said they must trust their partner.

As previously noted, a few of the women studied could enjoy supersex during a one-night stand or with a partner who was not their "soul mate." But the vast majority spoke of the importance of a special and loving relationship. "I must have deep feelings of love for the man. After that, the mood just comes," said Rhonda, thirty-two. Another woman says, "I need to have trust in a man and in myself in order to let go, and for me that only comes with love."

Often these women will choose a period of celibacy rather than get sexually involved with a partner they don't deeply love. Leslie, twenty-seven, who reports having to be "passionately attracted to a man" before she can reach supersexual peaks, says, "For the past six months, I have taken a vow of celibacy, and it has really helped me understand how the feelings I enjoy during sex can be heightened in the rest of my life. I do a lot of mountain biking and rock climbing—all those activities that put my body in harmony with nature—and I've found that sometimes just sitting quietly by a brook can be more incredible than orgasm. I feel a little calmer in nature. Compared to sex, the adrenaline high is not as exhilarating. But the feelings are still fantastic."

Wanda, forty-three and a lesbian, says, "To fully connect with someone, I have to feel a deep bond with her—a deep, almost unconditional love." Another lesbian, Sharine, recalls that after one supersexual moment during which she almost "blacked out," she was so profoundly moved that "I just broke down emotionally. I was crying, crying, crying while she was holding me and it was like I couldn't hold her close enough. I could never have done that if I didn't feel deeply loved. It was like—oh, wow! It was so beautiful. It felt wonderful being able to let go like that."

A few women draw a distinction between being "in love" and sharing a warm loving-kindness. Claire speaks for several supersexual women when she says, "I don't have to be 'in love,' but the person does have to be someone with whom I can feel comfortable genuinely being myself."

Joe, Catherine's partner, explains, "Part of loving is building something together. And making love is something of the same thing. It's not a feeling of who's got more power, but that we're both swimming in the same direction. Great sex depends upon the relationship as much as it does the activity you're engaged in."

Love, of course, has never been fully defined, even by poets who have spent whole lifetimes trying to do so. But fortunately, we needn't define love to know it. When asked which qualities they must have in a loving relationship to reach sexual ecstasy the women in our study were surprisingly clear: a sense of safety and a feeling of acceptance. Of course feeling accepted and safe are arrived at through one's own efforts, but the partner's willingness to nurture the process is important.

A Sense of Safety

A woman creates her own sense of safety by being clear—both in her own mind and with her partner—about what pleases and hurts her. As she learns to value her inner signals and gains confidence about setting limits with partners who may mistreat her, she is more able to embrace supersexual joy. She learns to discriminate between times when it's okay, or not okay, to be vulnerable. So, while it's true that some partners are safer and more respectful than others, a sense of safety is basically a feeling a woman creates for *herself* by refusing to become involved with someone who will hurt her.

Before she began enjoying supersex, Penny went through a period when she felt very "used" by the men she dated. Her first intercourse (*not* a supersexual moment) was at age eighteen in Australia with a man who swore she was the woman of his dreams. He promised he'd soon move to the United States so that they could be together. But a few weeks after Penny returned to the States, he stopped writing; when she realized she hadn't been special to him after all, she became hurt and depressed. Then she met Scott, twenty-eight, a very sensitive lover. Penny describes how their bond of trust developed:

> From the moment we began dating, it was a really special relationship because I didn't feel any sexual pressure from him. I didn't feel as if I had to have sex with him just to make the relationship last. I probably would have had sex with him on our first date because I was still a little unstable. But he was the one who said, "You're not ready yet. When the time comes, you'll know. We have plenty of time." So we became friends first, and it was a very comfortable relationship right from the beginning. He took that pressure off.
>
> The first time we made love it was so beautiful I can't even put it into words. We'd had a great dinner and we'd

spent the night together just talking. Then we started kissing and one thing led to another and I said, "Scott, I'm ready. I think this is it, I'm ready." And he didn't ask, "Are you sure?" He just looked at me, and he knew. He went really slow and was very considerate of my feelings. He was very sweet. It was just great. Afterwards, I cried, and I didn't know why. But he said, "It's okay, you can cry." I just felt so accepted for who I was and how I felt. It was very special.

The first time Penny supersexually connected with Scott was about a year later.

It just happened one day when we were very relaxed. I forgot about what we were doing or where we were and lost myself in the moment. I thought, "You don't have to prove yourself anymore. He loves you for who you are." It was nice to know he loved my body, that he loved what I looked like. I also felt secure in the relationship and in myself.

A Sense of Acceptance

For women, feeling physically attractive is often central to opening to love. In a society where they are frequently held up to impossible standards of beauty, many women feel they are not acceptable unless they are a perfect size 8, cellulite-free, and look like the models in *Vogue*. For these women, learning to feel comfortable, more secure, and less shameful of their bodies is important to enjoying sexuality. Knowing that your partner finds you attractive is helpful, but external reassurance is rarely enough. Supersexual women have learned, through a variety of ways, to become less self-critical and more self-affirming. Some of them have learned this through formal therapy, self-help books such as *Bodylove* by psychologist Rita Freedman, or using some other cognitive-behavioral approach designed to stop negative thinking and replace it with loving affirmations.

Five foot eight and about 130 pounds, with dark curly hair and large brown eyes, Kimberly has the kind of classic beauty immortalized by Greek scupltors. It's easy to see why she was hired as a makeup consultant by a well-known department store chain. Yet here's how she describes her "imperfect" body and her transition toward self-acceptance with her partner's help:

I've always had, not a *problem* with my body, but I've never thought of myself as perfect either. I've always thought of myself as needing to lose ten pounds or so. But since day one, Luke has always told me how much he likes my figure. He likes bigger, full-figured girls. I know I'm not fat, but I have "breeder hips," as my brother says. I'm not like a Paulina type. [She's referring to ultra-thin model Paulina Porizkova.] So ever since Luke told me how much he loves looking at me, I thought, "That's cool, because now I don't have to worry about him going after the Paulina types." Not that he would, but you know that's always in the back of your mind when a skinny, good-looking woman walks by. You know, everybody turns and looks at her and the first thing that goes through your mind is, "Well, she's skinnier than me." So when he said, "I love your legs," I thought, "Oh, wow, I don't have to lose ten pounds for this man to think I'm pretty." During sex, when I'm lying there naked and he says, "I just love your body," it helps me relax. I mean, he's got his arrogance and his selfishness, but he lets me be the person I've always known I could be. His favorite line is "Just let me love you."

The first time I had a peak sexual experience—my first awesome orgasm—was when he took the time to explore every part of my body. We were in a room in his brother's house and we just started kissing and hugging. We kiss a lot, which I love. Kissing is my favorite sport. So he just pushed me gently back on the bed. I could smell the pillow and I could smell him. You know, some women say they like for a man to be all freshly showered and clean when they make love. Well, I just love his smell when he's come home from a hard day's work. He's a landscaper and as he's lifting a lot of stuff he's sweating, and I just love that manly smell. As he kissed me all over and stroked me with his hand, he would say, "Tell me when to stop," and I would say, "Oooh, don't stop, that's good." [Laughs joyously.] We were just really playful that day, tumbling and flipping over, all sorts of fun things.

I'd had several orgasms when, at one point, I was on top of him. I looked down at him and just by the way he was looking at me, I had another one. Before in sex, I was always holding back. But for some reason, his staring into my eyes right at that moment took the last bit of resistance from me. I felt good being looked at that way—good about myself. Then he started moving under me, and I kept having orgasms, and he started moving me back and forth, back and forth on top of him. Suddenly, it was like everything—my feelings, my mind—were closing in and all I could feel was these great waves of energy radiating up through my whole body. I couldn't hear anything, I couldn't see anything. The orgasm started at my genitals and went clear up to my head. It was like the vibrations, the contractions were happening *inside* my head. All my senses were shut down, and I think for a minute I passed out. I just fell over. I'm glad I didn't fall into space. [Laughs.] And suddenly I could hear Luke saying, "Kim, Kim—are you okay?" And I just opened my eyes and went, "Whoa! What happened? We've gotta do that again because that was one singular feeling."

Trusting her partner completely often frees a woman to let go of more than sexual inhibitions. Since this super-sexual experience Kimberly has continued to let go of her unrealistic expectations for perfection. She says, "I may look at my body now and say, 'You've got to do more squats and get rid of that cellulite,' but I don't think of myself as ugly anymore."

Whereas some women need to accept themselves and feel accepted physically before they can experience the ultimate connection, others need to feel that their lovers respect their strength and independence. That's certainly a priority for Claire, who describes her special partner this way:

The man was an intellectual, yet couldn't hold a steady job. At the time of the affair, he was living in some make-shift, trailer-type home on the property of a professor for whom he did odd jobs.

I don't remember what we talked about, but I remember he was a very sensitive man and understood women very well. He had a lot of "feminine" traits. I have some "masculine" traits, which seem to turn some men off. But he wasn't biased against my strength; it wasn't an issue.

I am giving all this background because I think it is essential to the sexual experience. If I feel overpowered or used at all, I cannot enjoy the sex. All men I have especially enjoyed sex with—whether it was spontaneous sex or not—have been sensitive men who have stereotypically feminine traits and understand, accept, appreciate, and love the strength and power of a woman.

I don't remember the surroundings, except that we were in my bedroom. I don't remember if the light was on or off or what I was wearing. I only remember it was quiet and safe. I had no sense of our surroundings—there was only me, him, and the act.

During intercourse, I was only aware that he was pressing gently and firmly deep inside me. I didn't feel as if he was wanting to overpower me or even necessarily to fulfill his own physical urges. I felt, instead, as if he wanted to blend with me.

At one point during our lovemaking, I felt as though I was "on another plane." White light filled the blackness behind my eyelids. I felt as if I was in the womb, which was a translucent, comfortable, pliable eggshell. I heard sounds from outside the womb. I felt it was the voice of my father. I could feel loving feelings all around me, and I felt part of that love. I don't remember a physical orgasm, but a wonderful mental release—a rebirth and cleansing.

Though we've used this as an example of a woman's
need to have her strength respected, notice again how
many images of safety Claire weaves through her memories of this moment. From the quiet of the room to the
comfort of feeling enveloped in her mother's womb listening to her father's voice, feelings of warmth and
safety. For her, these were necessary ingredients to
supersex.

When the Partner Is Enjoying Supersex, Too

As a by-product of *genuinely* wanting to win a woman's
trust, these women's partners may greatly intensify their
own sexual pleasure.

David certainly has. A caterer who works weekends as
a musician in a jazz band, David has been married seven
years to Rose, the first woman he ever slept with and the
only one he ever loved. He rates his happiness with their
sex life as a 6 on a scale of 0 to 6 and explains why sex
with Rose is so sensational he can hardly find words to describe it. "The important thing when we're making love is
that I'm making love with *her*. With *her*. I'm not focusing
on what I've heard that having sex is supposed to be. Not
what it says you're supposed to do in any book or film that
I might have seen or read. I'm not imagining I'm having
sex with some woman I saw at work. You know what I
mean? It's so incredible because I'm totally focused on
her—nobody else."

David continues: "Some men think that once they've
been married for a few years, sex has to get dull, so they
have to fool around to get turned on again. I don't need another woman to get me excited because Rose is a different
woman every time we're together. Sometimes she likes

sex hot and hard, sometimes she likes it soft and gentle,
sometimes she's playful ... and she's *all* these women."
So what's going through David's mind while they're
making love?

I don't want to come across sounding mystical, but it's almost like I'm transported to a metaphysical realm. Sometimes long before orgasm, I see the color red—like an
infrared wash over everything. When it's red, I always
sense that we're very much together. Our minds stay very,
very locked together throughout the whole act. Sometimes
I feel like I'm ascending above us, and I get these real
flashes of intense energy and brightness.

And what's Rose doing while David is floating and seeing red? She's tumbling through space. "It's like being
tumbled in a wave. I don't know which way is up or down.
Right before I have an orgasm, I fall down somewhere. In
fact, that's usually the last thing I say before I come: 'I'm
going to fall, Dave.' "

Another man who's enjoying supersex is Felicia's lover
Jason, a man she describes as her soulmate and the first
"fully conscious partner" she's ever known. Asked what
she means by "fully conscious," she replies, "He just really
pays attention to our relationship. When I'm so preoccupied I'm *not* paying attention, he emotionally seeks me.
Yesterday, for example, I was racing around because I was
rushing to go out for a day of shopping. I'd given him a
dozen little quick kisses as I ran in and out of the room.
But suddenly he took hold of me, pressed me to him, and
kissed me. I'm not saying he *forced* me to kiss him. He just
gently pressed me to him until I made the emotional connection. And I went, 'Oh! Good morning!' It was like I
woke up to him. He has that capacity to know when I'm
not fully connected with him, and he *seeks* connection."

During lovemaking, she says, "I never feel manipulated or pressed by him at all. But—how can I say it?—often when I'm with him, it's almost as though he *plays* my body like an instrument. The rhythm is always right for me. He senses me. And when he finally enters me and we're rhythmic together, it's as if my consciousness becomes more enlarged." A private man, Jason declined to be interviewed, so we can't describe one of his specific supersexual moments for you. But Felicia says, "He's definitely transcending with me—we often talk about it."

Joe *was* willing to share what's happening to him while Catherine is lost in light:

> There are many variations on what people consider love. We've reached that deepest level where I feel we're true soulmates. When I touch her, it's almost as if I can feel what she's feeling. I've never been able to do this with any other woman. Sex with Catherine is what I would think a drug experience is like, but it's much finer and purer than that. I can go on for hours. It's a hard thing to describe. It's so enveloping. It's a lot like I'm charged with electricity. It's a very weird sensation—almost as if I'm leaving my body. But not like a near-death experience. It's like all my muscle fibers are firing until I feel like I'm going to explode. Then I do. There's a world of difference between making love and having sex, and I feel like I'm making love now. It's the closest I've ever come to a religion.

Just as supersexual women usually rate their first intercourse low on the pleasure scale, Joe says his first intercourse at age sixteen didn't begin to approach the ecstasy he's now feeling at age thirty-nine. "Back then I was just looking for immediate gratification," he recalls. "I had no concept of what it meant to form a real relationship. I didn't know what the hell I was doing."

Does Supersex Make a Relationship Perfect?

Listening to couples like these, one might wonder, does sexual ecstasy automatically lead to a perfect relationship? Unfortunately, no. Supersexual women struggle with all the romantic problems many women battle—from too much emotional distance in their marriages to too little commitment from the men they're dating. Four months after our interview, for example, Felicia and Jason broke up. Why? Fully conscious or not, he wouldn't marry her. With the wounds of his previous marriage still unhealed, he was unable to make the commitment. That's not to say this romance has definitely ended. During the course of our investigation, Catherine and Joe also broke up. Still married to another woman at the time, Joe went back to his wife for several months. Now, after his divorce, he and Catherine are back together and planning to marry.

Sexual ecstasy can certainly be one element in a happy love affair or marriage. But when problems erupt—as they can between any two people—supersex won't necessarily smooth out the frustrations. Kelly, a forty-six-year-old personnel manager, has been enjoying supersex with her husband for more than twenty-five years. Yet she says, "There are days when we're more in tune than others. You know, some days I absolutely *hate* him. I'm angry, we're not in sync, and sex goes to pot."

Helene, the forty-three-year-old piano instructor who during her very best sexual encounters sees colors like gold, white, and orange, is presently quite angry with her hard-driving executive husband of twenty years. "He really externalizes his anger, and I end up the scapegoat," she says. "So when he's tense, which is most of the time, he just can't relax and open up to me." Even so, she can still sometimes immerse herself so completely in her own pleasure that she can reach supersexual peaks. But she adds that their present marital strife makes sex a lot less satisfying than it used to be. "It's very hard for Hugh [her husband] to connect on a deep heart-to-heart level. I go through periods where I can overcome that and other times when I get fairly impatient with him. The more self-centered he is, the more boring sex becomes for me. Part of myself becomes a bit guarded. I can't let go as completely."

Yet despite her frustrations, Helene has chosen to see her husband's problems not as a personal attack upon her, but as an opportunity for her own spiritual growth. Referring to a flirtation her husband recently had with a student half his age, she says philosophically, "He's a wonderful man, really. This is just like a stage he's going through. I believe that if you're really working on yourself, if you're on a spiritual path and trying to raise your consciousness, you're going to be tested like this. But if I just sit around and blame him, then I'm not focusing on the problems in myself that I can work on, too. I think his struggles can teach me more understanding and compassion."

Rather than dwelling on the ways her husband is making her miserable, Helene has learned how to rise above her problems. One pleasure for her is yoga. Explaining what she enjoys most about it, she says: "I love that sense of going beyond time and space. Some good friends of mine started meditating about the same time I did. But when they would have real intense experiences, it would just scare them. They found that sense of going beyond boundaries uncomfortable. But it's not unpleasant to me. I love it. As a teenager, I used to have that same feeling while surfing—that feeling of letting go and becoming totally at one with nature, with something beyond myself. I think when you give yourself these experiences, you can bring them to the rest of your life and gain a deeper appreciation for the ups and downs."

Why doesn't Helene divorce Hugh rather than put up with his anger? After all, isn't the goal of life to be happy? She has chosen to stay with him. What we realized is that Helene isn't suffering in the same way other women in her situation might because she regularly takes time out to transcend her problems by focusing inward—the same practice that can lead to great sexual fulfillment.

∽ CHAPTER 8 ∾

Courageously
Opening to Life

*It costs so much to be a full human being that
there are few who have the love and courage to
pay the price. One has to abandon altogether
the search for security and reach out to the risk
of living with both arms. One has to embrace
life like a lover.*

—novelist Morris West

Women are reaching sexual peaks not because they're un-
commonly beautiful or have managed to find just the right
erotic position or the perfect partner. What they are experiencing sexually is a reflection of the courageous ways
they've chosen to open themselves up to life. More important, our research has convinced us that each and every
one of us has the capacity to reach this uppermost level of
sexual functioning. *Achieving one's full sexual potential is
an ability available to any of us willing to live courageously
enough to pursue it.*

Yet even as we say this, we know that the ecstasy of
supersex cannot be pursued—it can only ensue. For
supersex is like happiness: the minute we aim consciously
for it, it eludes us. You can't *make* a peak sexual experience happen, but you can set up all the conditions so that
one is more *likely* to happen. In the end, supersex comes
to us not as a result of trying to force it, but as a by-
product of getting in touch with the true self.

Supersexual women have found the courage to listen to themselves. By learning to trust and respond to their inner pleasure signals, they come to know what they most value and which experiences most deeply satisfy and enrich them. It could be reading a poem with their morning coffee; sunbathing nude in the backyard; deeply inhaling the fresh air after a spring rain; or savoring one exquisite chocolate truffle. Treating themselves daily to such pleasures helps keep them centered and whole. Danielle adores the fresh, springlike scent of her lover's body (to her, he smells "like lilacs, but not quite as sweet"). Constance loves burying her face in the delicate skin of her lover's neck ("it's so smooth and soft, it feels like the skin of a doe").

It may be tempting to view these women's approach to life as self-absorbed in a hedonistic way, a bit like the philosophy, "If it feels good, do it." But it would be a great mistake to dismiss these women as hedonists living only for the moment or looking out just for themselves. They're simply taking the time and making the disciplined effort to enhance the inner quality of their lives.

What is this "true self" with which supersexual women have gotten so in touch? It's the most basic part of our being—that loving self that existed in us before we began narrowing down our options and restricting our opinions about who we are. The true self or "real self" was defined by Karen Horney as a "central inner force—central to all—equated with healthy integration and harmonious coherence . . . a source of constructive growth, spontaneity, energy, interest, clarity, depth of feeling, and resourcefulness" (From *Neurosis and Human Growth*, W.W. Norton, 1950). When you're living according to the highest values of the true self, you're expressing your essential nature—the person you were meant to be. Observe a baby only a few months old and you'll see the earliest stirrings of the formative true self in action. Although the environment begins to "shape" a baby's responses right from birth, the infant is essentially unschooled in how she's "supposed" to respond to an engrossing sight, aroma, taste, touch, or sound. A baby's gaze, her rapt attention, is transfixed by whatever captures her interest. There's something attractive in that spontaneity. Just notice the way people generally respond to infants. It's not unusual to see people smiling at babies—engaging them—drawn to that light behind an infant's eyes.

What is it about a newborn baby that resonates in many of us? Perhaps, in the unbridled joy with which a baby addresses life, we can see the essence of ourselves, that spark of divinity, the seed of "perfection." It is a similar spark or essence that supersexual women report when experiencing their most transcendent moments.

But what happens to this true self as we grow and develop? It often becomes constrained. The limiting self is that collection of opinions we have learned to believe about ourselves. Developing a limiting self, of course, is a necessary step in human growth. To form an identity, a person has to define who she is and what she values. For example, she may come to think of herself as a person who likes carrots, but hates peas; loves reading but hates math; or can tell jokes that make her friends laugh. The things you believe about yourself create your reality. You may come to believe that you're not talented in art, have an average intellect, or that you're a poor athlete. You may believe that you have a "selfish nature" just because someone proclaimed it at your sixth birthday (when you asked for the piece of birthday cake with the large icing flower). Throughout childhood we are subjected to a plethora of parental and societal voices saying, *"Stop laughing so loudly—you'll wake your sister! Stop running so fast—you'll get hurt! Stop daydreaming and pay attention! Don't touch yourself 'down there,' it's not nice [when it feels nice]! What are you sad about—there's nothing to be sad about! What are you afraid of—there's nothing to be afraid of! What are you happy about—there's nothing to be happy about!"* As the opinions of how we "should" feel clash with how we genuinely feel, self-doubts may creep in about the validity of our inner signals. Step by step and year after year we may begin to choose what *others* define as "good" or "bad" and to discount our own direct experiences. As we deny our inner reality and allow it to become buried beneath a chorus of voices, our own voice—the voice of the true self—may speak more and more softly until some of us can no longer hear it at all.

This is not to suggest that intuition is supreme or that all societal teachings are restrictive, but that we should recognize the wisdom waiting inside.

How does the limiting self express itself during sex? You can tell when this part of you is busily at work when you find yourself judging, critiquing, stepping outside your immediate present experience. Such thoughts as "It's selfish to think about my own pleasure during sex—I should be thinking more about my partner's pleasure;" "I shouldn't fantasize about the ocean or about a favorite sexual fantasy while making love—that's abnormal;" or "I should come more quickly during intercourse, before my partner does—I don't want him to think he has 'premature ejaculation;' " are a product of the limiting self and when you limit yourself, you inevitably limit your sexual potential.

Honesty, Empowerment, and Choice

In our quest to uncover the keys to supersexual response, we studied the personality characteristics of our subjects in depth. The written 300-question personality inventory they took, coupled with in-depth interviews, reveals that high absorbers share a remarkable number of qualities. Three of the most critical attributes related to becoming supersexual are self-empowerment, honesty, and the courage to go her own way.

The "findings" that follow were taken fairly directly from an item analysis of the personality inventory. This material is not presented as a standard for behavior, but merely suggests the pattern of responses in our sample. Because such similar qualities emerged they struck us as significant. However, possessing (or not possessing) these qualities does not necessarily predict or preclude supersexual experience. These characteristics represent a majority of responses and are intended as absolutes for *all* supersexual women.

Honesty

Supersexual women tend to be frank, trustworthy, and forthright—both with themselves and with others. This honesty does not come from a strict moral code set up by others, but rather from self-knowledge. Supersexual women seldom report feeling vengeful when "wronged." When unjustly criticized, they don't allow their anger to consume them, but find an appropriate way to express and handle their feelings. According to their answers on the personality inventory, they consider themselves fair.

Most supersexual women report being attracted to excellence: they take pride in their work, and strive to be the best they can be—but not at the expense of the overall quality of their lives. They consider the warmth of being in a group of friends one of their most satisfying experiences, saying that without close relations with others their lives would be far less worthwhile.

During our interviews with them, supersexual women appeared to be very open, nonjudgmental, and truthful in their responses. Are these women truly as open and honest as they appear? Our findings suggest that they are. One objective indication of this conclusion comes from the personality inventory. The test contains several "validity scales" that measure the accuracy of their responses. For example, in some cases the same question is asked twice, but the wording differs. Other statements are designed to see whether the test-taker will claim to possess an unlikely virtue: someone who asserts she has *never* been envious of anyone or that her opinions are *always* "completely reasonable" is probably stretching the truth. We had decided that if any of the women interviewed were later shown to be fudging on the written personality test we would exclude her from the study. But not one woman reporting a supersexual experience had to be eliminated from our research sample. According to the validity measures, these women were being candid.

Supersexual women have made a loving, courageous choice: they have looked deeply inside themselves to examine their strengths and limitations. They're more confident of their own views. They are also trusting of their own judgments and first impressions. When they receive messages from their unconscious—messages that have been variously called intuitions, sudden insights, or hunches—they use them to enrich their interpersonal relationships. As a result, they're usually excellent at reading situations and people. If they're deceived or mistaken in their judgment, it's usually not for very long. The clarity and honesty they demand from themselves make it easier for them to perceive honesty in others. This process of self-discovery, introspection, and self-acceptance is ongoing and never-ending. Supersexual women demonstrate the courage to persevere in their own psychological growth and development.

Self-Empowerment

Even when life isn't going their way, supersexual women have learned how to empower themselves. Some of these women were battered as children, grew up in poverty, or were deaf from birth. But whatever the realities of their lives, they have chosen to open up to the joys of living rather than close themselves off. They're not afraid to be childlike at times—to let their minds wander in a pleasant daydream, to become lost in a science-fiction novel, or to revel in an imaginative fantasy. Curious, creative, and spontaneous, they're ready to engage with life and with what gives them pleasure, whether it's running a marathon, sleeping out under the stars, checking into a four-star hotel, riding in a hot-air balloon, or starting up their own business. Thus, despite difficulties they may face, these women say they're usually happy to be alive. Many of us let the problems, trials, and stresses we have to face dominate our lives. But supersexual women have learned that even under the most difficult circumstances they still have a choice: they can choose the attitude they'll take toward any given situation—promising or problematic.

In his classic book *Man's Search for Meaning*, in which he described his experiences as a Jew in a Nazi concentration camp, psychoanalyst Viktor Frankl wrote that even in the most brutal of circumstances, he and his fellow prisoners sometimes knew moments of serenity—when, for example, they vividly recalled a loved one's face or caught a glimpse of some beauty in nature, such as a common tree or a sunrise. "We who lived in concentration camps," Frankl wrote, "can remember the men who walked through the huts comforting others, giving away their last piece of bread. They may have been few in number, but they offer sufficient proof that everything can be taken from a man but one thing: the last of the human freedoms—to choose one's attitude in any given set of circumstances, to choose one's own way."

Supersexual women have chosen their own way. By directing their attention toward those experiences that most please them—and controlling the attitude they will take toward any given situation—they have learned to enhance the quality of their lives. One of our interviewees, Jane, age forty-six, told us that as a child, she was slapped by her father almost daily. "He would lash out suddenly for the slightest provocation. I became so accustomed to being hit that I learned to block out the sting and 'turn myself off.' " When her father realized the beatings were not reaching her, he resorted to name-calling and emotional abuse. "That didn't work either, because I just tuned him out of my head. Sometimes he'd go on for what seemed to be hours, but I'd be safe inside of myself somewhere. . . . I'd say to myself, 'He's not right. I'm a good person.' Or I'd just construct my favorite fairy-tale fantasy or imagery of a completely safe place—usually the hollow of a big elm tree."

Some people who "separate themselves from reality," as Jane did, wind up splitting off parts of themselves in an attempt to cope with their trauma. Psychologists call this phenomenon *dissociation.* Later in life, such women often report that they have "no feeling" during sex because they've learned to turn off their feelings. The supersexual women we studied, however, have used dissociation in a positive, healthy way to tune out others' negative opinions about them and to immerse themselves in pleasure or comforting imagery.

In many ways, supersexual women resemble those people psychologist Al Siebert has called "survivors." Interviewing hundreds of people who have successfully endured all kinds of hardships, Siebert has found that the survivor personality contains a number of qualities supersexual women share. Among the most striking parallels are:

- an ability to become so deeply engrossed in an activity that you lose all track of time and what's happening around you
- an active imagination, expressed by daydreaming, fantasizing, and conversations with yourself
- a recognition of intuition and a kind of inner awareness as a valid source of knowledge
- an ability to stay positive and optimistic in the face of adversity
- a talent for being able to absorb all kinds of experiences—good and bad—and allow the self to develop within them
- the feeling that you're gaining wisdom and enjoying life more as you grow older

Notably, these are the same characteristics New Haven cancer surgeon Dr. Bernie Siegel has observed in people who survive cancer despite the odds against them.

A surprising number of supersexual women *are* survivors: of incest, rape, battering, alcoholic families, and other abuse. As you'll see in Chapter 9, one woman survived breast cancer. Rather than becoming embittered or traumatized by these events to the point where they can't function, these women have often turned their pain into a positive vehicle for self-growth. As Carl Jung said, "Neurosis is always a substitute for legitimate suffering." Rather than evading suffering, these women face worries, pain, and fears squarely and use pain as an opportunity to grow.

The Courage to Choose Their Own Way

In our society we're treated to many simplistic formulas for making sex great.

Every day we're inundated with spoken and unspoken myths about what it means to be sexy and how we can make our erotic lives more intense: *If sex has become dull, you just need to find a new erotic position. If your lovemaking has lost its pizzazz, you only need to surprise your partner with some hot lingerie or make an appointment for sex. When it comes to your love life, great sex will be yours if you'll only follow this or that prescription.* While such suggestions can often be helpful, the road to supersex cannot be found by listening to external prescriptions. Achieving true sexual ecstasy involves not only listening to outside authorities, but mapping your own route to pleasure.

Supersexual women intuitively know this. By taking the time to listen to their inner signals, they have learned to trust their own authority and look to their own hearts for guidance. Many supersexual women *have* found guidance through friendships, self-help books, or formal therapy, however, they tend to be a group of women who are especially sensitive and tuned-in to their own inner signals. They have taken the time to listen to these signals and acknowledge them. They have learned to trust their own inner guidance to lead them to what they need from the outside world.

One outward sign of their unconventional attitude toward life is the way they tend to approach religion and spirituality. Before she had what she calls her "spiritual-psychological-sexual awakening," one woman says, she went to church in a routine way every Sunday only to please her parents. Now she goes only about once a month to take communion and feel a oneness with God. She regrets, however, that the reading of the weekly bulletins and other talking that goes on in church often get in the way of her ability to feel the deeply focused kind of spiritual connection she usually experiences in nature. She says, "As I've told my pastor, I sometimes think the most meaningful way to conduct a church service would be for everyone to sit in the pews in absolute silence and meditate for two hours while the organ softly plays."

By going their own way even at the risk of seeming unconventional, supersexual women have become what one of them called "independently capable." During our talks with these women, we were frequently impressed by the aptness of this phrase: supersexual women are, indeed, independently capable. They know their own minds and are decisive and forceful enough to go after what they want.

Is it a paradox that women who can connect at such a profound level with their partners so frequently describe themselves as independent and self-sufficient? No. We found in our research women who comfortably contain many opposites within their personalities. Supersexual women are both sociable and introspective, impulsive and cautious, intuitive and logical, shy and forceful, connected to others and independent, able to control and to let go. As human beings, we all contain these opposites within us. But because they see the gray areas as well as the black and white choices, and are so in touch with themselves, supersexual women can embrace seemingly disparate aspects of their personalities. They have found what George Leonard has called "the courage to lead an essentially unpredictable life."

Supersexual women have a clarity of mind and spirit as well as a subtle charismatic quality. Many of the supersexual women we studied knew they had this charisma, but seemed genuinely baffled by it. Asked if she aspires to power, for example, Felicia replied, "Well, I've always had a lot of personal power. I don't know why. It just sits around me. Sometimes I find it a bit unnerving that people listen to me as easily as they do. A lot of people see me as authoritative. Some almost seem to follow me as if I'm a Pied Piper, and it perplexes me. I can't understand why they look to me for answers." By going their own way, the women who emerged as supersexual naturally exude an air of having discovered a "secret" many of us long to share.

The abilities to go beyond the limited self, see her private reality clearly, and then choose to go her own way are among the most important qualities a woman must develop before she can reach supersexual bliss. Why? Because our expectations of what's *possible* limit our capabilities. *To become supersexual, a woman may have to transcend many of the ways she has been culturally "trained" to think of sex.*

At this point, you may be thinking, "Well, it's fine that these women have all of these virtues. It sounds as though to have supersex, you just have to be a good person, and I am a good person. But I don't feel any closer to supersex than I did before." In the chapters that follow, you'll find out much more about what brings women of all ages and stages to supersexual levels of enjoyment, and how to begin—or continue—that journey yourself.

❧ PART II ❧

Becoming Supersexual

Are you up to your destiny?
　　　　　　　　—Shakespeare, *Hamlet*

(

⧆ CHAPTER 9 ⧆

Those Who Learn Young

children guessed (but only a few)

—e.e. cummings,
"anyone lived in a pretty how town"

When we began this investigation, we halfway expected to find a progression in female sexual development much like the model of adult development Gail Sheehy described in *Passages,* in which women would achieve one set of skills or level of sexual awareness in their twenties, another perhaps by age thirty-five, still another in their forties, and so forth. In other words, we thought the route to one's full sexual potential might be marked by separate stages or passages—and at each passage we'd be called on to overcome certain milestones or accomplish specific tasks.

Instead, we found that the capacity for supersexual joy is not age-related. Some women have this ability in their teens and early twenties.

These "young absorbers," as we came to call them, were extraordinarily independent. They reported such experiences as traveling cross-country alone at age ten, going to Europe alone at sixteen, or taking care of their basic financial needs from the time they were thirteen or fourteen.

How did they manage so early to achieve levels of sexual wholeness some women seek their entire lives? The most obvious theory, of course, would be that they must all have come from sexually open, happy, supportive families, and indeed some of them did.

When Supersex Begins with Loving Parents

Nicole is an easygoing college freshman with a mane of thick dark hair and a warm Mona Lisa smile. She is supersexual at nineteen and credits her parents with her ability to choose kind, caring men. She says, "None of my boyfriends has ever pressured me to have sex, because I choose them that way. I don't choose a guy just by how he looks, and I would never pick up a man in a bar. I watch a man to see how he treats his friends and his family. I want to touch a man not for his face, not for his body, but for his soul. I think even without them explicitly telling me what to look for, I've learned a lot from my parents about how to choose men who will care about and respect me. I see the love my dad shows for my mom, and I will never settle for anything less than that."

At fourteen, Nicole got a job in a yogurt shop because she wanted to earn her own money. In four years, she had saved enough from her work and gifts from relatives that when her mother admired a diamond ring in a jewelry store, Nicole recalls proudly, "I just wrote out a check and said, 'It's yours.' "

Nicole's mother is a strong, confident woman who says she and her husband both value their daughter's independence. She says, "Nicole was always strong-willed, and sometimes I admit wishing she had been easier to raise. But that's the way she is. I always tried to accept her for what she is—to be not just her mother, but also her friend. You can't change people. Why would you want to? Certainly, I tried to teach Nicole commonsense rules of right and wrong—simple rules like stealing is bad. But if I like her hair cut short and she prefers to wear it long, why should I insist she do it my way? I admire differences in people. Nature is one of the most beautiful things on earth, simply because it's so varied." She then gives Nicole her highest compliment. "My daughter," she says proudly, "is an original."

Perhaps the most we can say about Nicole's parents is that they did not get in her way: they seem to have established an atmosphere of warmth and respect around their daughter that nurtured supersexual needs.

Nicole's parents made her feel it was okay to take responsibility for her life.

When Supersex Emerges Without Loving Parents

Certainly a happy childhood is preferable to a troubled one in any case. Yet it would be a great mistake to conclude from this that if you happen to have had an unhappy childhood you're destined never to reach supersexual peaks. There is no hard-and-fast cause-and-effect chain operating here.

Brett, who is supersexual at age twenty, came from a divorced family. When she was young, Brett lived for several years with her father, whose rages terrified her. When she went to live with her mother at thirteen, she was repeatedly told what an "awful child" she was. "She constantly told me I was never going to do anything with my life. She put me down all the time. Then my stepfather decided I was not part of his family and they both disowned me." Her mother often refused to speak to her for months at a time. Brett found consolation in her best friend, Tim—a boy she'd known all her life. When she was sixteen, Tim was killed in a car wreck. Thus, at twenty, Brett has known more sorrow than many people experience in a lifetime. Yet she describes herself as "a survivor." According to her answers on the written personality test, she is optimistic about her future, and is not cynical, bitter, or manipulative. On the contrary, she's a socially astute, honest, well-adjusted young woman who fits the profile of wholeness we described in Chapter 6. You might say that Brett is using "denial" to cope with her feelings, or that she has learned to reframe problems as opportunities for growth. We feel the latter is more accurate.

You may recall that her first intercourse was the unpleasant encounter on the fourteenth hole of the golf course you read about earlier. And yet here's how she describes the fourth time she made love:

It was in his brother's Jeep in January with the top down. It was freezing, but it was wonderful. I don't know what it was about Chuck, but from the first time he kissed me, I just melted. I just got so excited, I said to myself, "Ooooh, boy. I'm going to get myself in trouble." [Laughs lightly.] I would do anything for him. We had been at his house watching a movie in which Kevin Costner had sex with a girl in a Jeep. And I was just watching this movie, thinking, "Oh boy, that's what *I* want to do!" So after the movie, it was about eleven o'clock at night, and I said, "Let's take the Jeep out." We went to this big mall in his town. It was completely deserted, and we just parked the car in the lot and had sex right there. It was beautiful, just beautiful. I was so happy I thought I would burst. It was like I left my body and I was watching myself. It was so weird. And I saw white. I felt like I was in heaven. I had never felt like that before in my life. It was beautiful, beautiful. It was just great.

Whereas Nicole got a job at fourteen because she wanted to, Brett had to became financially self-sufficient at thirteen.

She says, "My mother never helped me out financially. From the time I was thirteen, I used the money I earned from baby-sitting to buy my own shampoo, clothes, school supplies—everything I needed except food." Yet rather than blaming her parents or fate for her situation, Brett accepted this responsibility. "It was no big deal," she says, shrugging. "I *liked* taking care of myself. It made me stronger."

Many women don't become introspective enough to experience supersex until they're thirty, forty, or older. Women like Nicole and Brett, however, learned very early in life who they were, what genuinely mattered to them (as opposed to what others said was important), and how to stay in touch with their deepest feelings.

We'll now examine some key ways they did this. But as you're reading, remember it's not only *they* who can become this empowered. The choices these women made— even as children—are continually open to us all.

They Spent Time in Silent Solitude

When we seek clues to understanding how these young women became independently capable so early in life, we find that nearly all describe themselves as quiet, reflective kids who spent a great deal of time in solitude.

Moira, a twenty-three-year-old dance teacher who has felt supersexual for five years, says, "As a child, I spent hours on end alone in my room coloring, playing with my toys, and reading. Today, when I really need time out, I take it. Sometimes I'll take an hour or two, sometimes it's a couple of days." What does she do during these solitary times? "Nothing. I don't watch television. I don't read. I just kind of float free and get back in touch with myself."

During their time alone as children, these women often enjoyed peak moments which seemed to foreshadow the supersexual bliss they would enjoy as adults. Kiana, age twenty-seven, recalls, "I was about five and outside on my swing set. All my brothers and sisters were at school, so I was home alone. It was a spring day, I had just learned the word *supercalifragilisticexpialidocious,* and I kept saying that word over and over to myself as I stared up into the sky. Suddenly it was like I just flew into the sky and was lost in the bright, swirling clouds. I've never had that exact experience again, but I've had other experiences, especially in spring, when I'll hear an airplane flying overhead and it will bring back that deep contented feeling of being lost in the clouds and the blue sky."

Some of these children used their quiet time alone to soothe themselves when they were in pain. "We had a very regular family, no substance abuse, no violence," Linda recalls. "But one tragedy I did have to face was the death of my mother, who died when I was fourteen. One thing I used to do to comfort myself was to go out to our backyard hammock. I would just swing for hours alone, becoming so mesmerized by the repetitive movement I'd lose all track of time. It was a way to be available to myself—a form of deepening self-reliance."

It's understandable why spending quiet time alone might have helped these young women establish their supersexual identity. Through the ages, religious orders from Carthusian monks to Quakers have considered silence a way to refine and deepen oneself. Marsha Sinetar described the benefits of silent solitude well in *Ordinary People as Monks and Mystics* when she wrote:

It is in silence that our reflective ability—and our need to reflect—is born. In silence we grow more aware: sounds, however distant, or the absence of them, bring out the hidden parts of our personality, triggering thoughts and various fleeting phenomena in our body and attention. In silence we perceive the ineffable, that which cannot be verbalized, cannot be made concrete. In silence and solitude our individuality is affirmed.

One woman we studied drew a clear distinction between being alone and enjoying solitude: "You can be alone, say, in the kitchen, running around like a madwoman cleaning up before company comes, or you can enjoy *solitude,* which involves quietly communing with yourself. There's nothing great about being alone; but in solitude I can hear my own voice again."

Leila, who has been deaf from birth, told us, "I try to help hearing people understand what silence means to me. People think when you're deaf, there's a void. But I tell them, no, no, no—it's just the opposite. To me, silence is truth. In the silence within, you'll find the whole universe. I tell people, 'You, too, have a powerful heart of silence in you.' If you can't hear it, it's only because the world is so full of noises."

They Frequently Read Fairy Tales

Time and again, supersexual women reported leading highly imaginative fantasy lives. They especially love fairy tales, and once they learned to read could become so wrapped up in a story they could lose themselves in it for hours. As children, they weren't simply good readers, they were *involved* readers. As they read, they would develop vivid images to go along with the story.

When describing one of her favorite books—J.R.R. Tolkien's classic fantasy *The Lord of the Rings,* one young woman who began enjoying supersex at nineteen says: "The scenes in Mirkwood are still intensely vivid to me. Even now, I can almost smell, feel, and see that forest. It smells musty and dank—like a cellar with a woodsy smell—and the air feels clammy and stuffy. All around me, the woods are so dark I almost can't make out the individual trees, and way high above, the leaves are blocking out all the light. Occasionally, if I'm lucky, a little beam of light manages to break through." Even though she read this book eight years ago, she describes the scene as if she personally journeyed through Mirkwood yesterday.

Leila recalls that reading provided a real awakening for her. "I didn't really understand the value of reading until I was fourteen years old. Then one day I picked up *Lord of the Flies,* and it was a real awakening for me. I don't know how to explain it—I can't put my feelings in words—but I achieved a new awareness. It was like a door opened and I walked into another realm of reality." Joe told us that since he has awakened to supersex, he also spends a lot more time reading.

What is it about reading stories—especially fairy tales— that helped these young women get in touch with themselves and become supersexual so young? Fairy tales help us develop vivid images and focus inward. To paraphrase Jung and Freud, fairy tales are like dreams in that they provide a direct route to our unconscious minds. In his book *Actual Minds, Possible Worlds,* eminent Harvard psychologist Jerome Bruner observes that there are two basic modes of thought: *scientific* thought, which is logical, linear, and rational, the kind of thinking we use to solve problems; and *narrative* thought, the language of fairy tales, myth, drama, and poetry. University of California psychiatrist Allan B. Chinen, who has compiled a book of fairy tales for adults in their middle years called *Once Upon a Midlife,* calls narrative thought "the stuff of the human soul." He cites a Hasidic proverb which says, "Give people a fact or an idea and you enlighten their minds; tell them a story and you touch their souls." Many psychotherapists and hypnotherapists use myths, metaphors, and fairy tales in their practices as a form of healing. By causing us to suspend logical thought, reading fairy tales and other stories seems to be one doorway to supersexual awareness.

They Explored Their Inner World by Daydreaming

Even as children, many of these women were mavericks. Despite their keen ability to concentrate in school, for example, they usually paid rapt attention only in those classes that *interested* them. If the teacher began to drone on or the coursework got dull, these girls were daydreaming or gazing idly out the window.

At a very early age, these young absorbers also learned that if they were feeling bad, they could use daydreams for a while to make themselves feel better. Thus, as young children, they learned that they were in charge of their own pleasure—that joy did not come from the outside, but from within.

Even though Nicole credits her parents for her cheerful disposition, for example, she says she can make *herself* happy by escaping from her problems whenever she chooses—a skill she learned in elementary school, when the other kids teased her. "That's when I learned to be somewhere else. When they teased me, I would just imagine that I wasn't there, that I was with people who were nice. Because of my mind, I would never let them get to me. If I'm feeling depressed, I'll sometimes take a 'mind walk' in the park: by feeling what it would be like to be in the park, it's as if I'm one hundred percent there. It's not that I step outside of reality. I just make reality nicer for myself, and I've always done that."

As children, many of us were told that daydreaming is

an impractical, "lazy" waste of time. Yet the vivid fantasy lives these women learned to develop as children seem to have benefited them later as adults and helped them become more immersed during lovemaking. In a study done by Wendy E. Stock and James H. Geer at the State University of New York at Stony Brook, most of the women who listened to a ten-minute erotic tape became sexually excited. But women who reported that they fantasized while masturbating became measurably more excited than those who seldom fantasized. The original research that inspired this book (Scantling, 1990) also found that women who enjoy sexual fantasy—and fantasize frequently—report more intense sexual arousal and sexual enjoyment during both masturbation and sex with a partner.

By letting their minds float free during vivid daydreams, these women even as children seemed to be developing a number of complex skills they would use as adults to block out distractions, heighten their concentration, increase their arousal, and enter new erotic dimensions.

So what does all this tell us about becoming supersexual at *any* age? We now know that women who reached this level in their development during their teens and twenties were not simply gifted or blessed. The lessons these women learned are all interconnected. Establishing a supersexual identity (finding out who you truly are) usually involves spending time in solitude. Taking time to reflect often leads to daydreaming. Through vivid daydreaming and reading, these young absorbers discovered they could develop and experience their inner worlds. And by transcending, they learned that true happiness comes not from what they own or what they do, but from who they are. For others, becoming supersexual takes more time: only as adults—if we make the right choices—do we learn the qualities these women garnered as children.

CHAPTER 10

Those Who Learn
Later in Life

*As Carl Jung observed, the most important
problems of life cannot be solved, but only
outgrown, and this outgrowing requires "a new
level of consciousness."*

—Frances Vaughan,
The Inward Arc

Life is forgiving. If we have lost touch with our deep inner
joy as children, we can reconnect with it as adults. Many
women who became supersexual later in life spoke of going through a kind of "awakening," after which they reported becoming more open to all of life's pleasures. This
awakening can occur at any age. But among the women interviewed, it usually occurred sometime between their late
twenties and early forties.

Women Who Experience a Sudden Insight

Many women in our study recall a peak experience that
transformed them. Kelly, who we met in Chapter 7,
gives a classic example of how a sudden near-death experience helped her develop a heightened sensitivity to life in
all of its intensity. Through an insightful peak experience

in her twenties, she reports becoming supersexual practically overnight:

> I had gone to the hospital to have a regular D & C and I ran into complications. I was right outside the recovery room, and I can remember asking the nurse to tell the doctor I was in a lot of pain, that she'd better tell him because this wasn't normal. Then they took me into surgery and I stopped breathing. I could feel myself going out of my body and looking down on what was happening. Then everything got very, very bright, and I can remember being in a meadow—a bright meadow. There were flowers. It was very warm, very sunny. I could hear birds and I was walking, walking along this path. Then my grandmother appeared. She had died a few years earlier and I had been very close to her. She came up to me and said, "Follow these flowers, and this path will take you back because it's not your time." And I came back. I remember coming back. It was dark— much darker—and I was in a lot of pain.
>
> Even though this happened over twenty years ago, it's still intensely vivid. You see, I *knew* I was there. I just *knew* I was there. I felt a sense of being rejuvenated, a euphoric joy.
>
> Since that time, I've just been so thankful to be alive. I can smell flowers more intensely. I'm more keenly aware of people, scenes, colors, noises. I just have a heightened sense of appreciation for life.

Almost immediately after this experience, Kelly's marriage—and the sex within her marriage—greatly improved. "Before that experience I was much more into myself, not as giving, more closed-off. But since that time, I'm not afraid to show my love. I now also know it's okay to have some really ecstatic sexual experiences." Asked to describe how sex has improved, Kelly replies, "I don't know if I've ever tried to put it into words, it's more of a feeling than a verbal experience. When we're making love,

I just feel a heightened sensitivity all over—warm, vital, and tingly. It's hard to describe, but it's like being aroused and at peace at the same time. It feels warm and safe, but it's also bright. There's almost an aura—a field of energy— around myself and my husband. It encompasses us both. The first time this happened, I thought it was because I'd almost died and I was just so happy to be alive. I figured that as time went on, sex would become more like the way it was before. But it's been over twenty years, and it hasn't lost that intensity."

Controlling and Letting Go

The journey to supersex requires that a woman take the responsibility for protecting herself and creating her own safety. She must take *control* over her life. But to become truly supersexual, she must learn to *let go*. The Buddha spent at least sixteen years of his life seeking enlightenment, but found it only when he stopped seeking and just let it come to him.

But isn't this a paradox—that to become supersexual, you must take control of your life right up to the point where you must let go? Not at all. It might help to think of controlling and letting go not as opposites, but as complements, as parts of the *same* continuum. Like this:

Letting Go	Control
Vulnerability...	Self-Protection,
Openness, Trust	Self-Assertion

Becoming supersexual requires learning to flow freely back and forth along this continuum, so you don't get trapped at either end. It's this ability that people are praying for in the well-known Serenity Prayer:

God, give me the serenity to accept the things I cannot change, the courage to change the things I can and the wisdom to know the difference.

In other words, allow me to flow freely between the two ends of this continuum: allow me to know when to control and when to let go. This is called the Serenity Prayer for good reason. Supersexual women *can* flow freely—and appropriately—along this continuum. They also inevitably report carrying within them a great inner peace.

Knowing when to let go—and perhaps more important, being *able* to let go fully—is the key capacity a woman must develop to achieve sexual ecstasy. And when she does let go, her sexual response often goes off the charts. She may see colors, fireworks, and sheets of white light or hear waves crashing, water rushing, and wind through the trees. She can float or soar to the stars. She becomes supersexual, and feels changed forever.

A Closer Look

Because supersexuality comes to most women over the course of many years, their memories can lack detail. When faced with the diagnosis of breast cancer, Lisa chose to confront her personal crisis with courage. She began to enjoy supersex shortly thereafter, and is able to articulate her transformation very clearly.

Two years after her double mastectomy, Lisa's doctor brought her some wonderful news. "He said, 'Lisa, we can't explain this, but we believe in miracles; your cancer has disappeared!' It was the turning point of my life."

Though she didn't know it at the time, Lisa was already far along the road to supersex. As you read the following interview, you'll notice that Lisa's attitudes have changed in many ways. Among them:

- She's much more in the moment—much more spontaneous.
- She has given up judgmental thoughts about pleasing her partner and how well she's "performing."
- She's not trying to control the experience. ("I just let go and go with the flow.")
- She asserts her own needs.
- She has turned her attention inward, to how she's feeling inside.
- She focuses less on needing things to be happy. Simple pleasures can fill her with delight. As she says, "I don't want to *have,* I want to *feel.*"

INTERVIEWER: *I'd like you to recall a very peak sexual moment, one you would describe as the best, and tell me about it.*

LISA: One of my best. Well, before I was more apt to please my partner than to focus on pleasing myself. I've let go of a lot of real heavy thoughts like "Is he having fun? Do I look okay?" Now I'm more in each moment. I just figure that whatever happens during sex will be O.K.

INT: *Tell me more about it.*

LISA: I'm often excited before we're even in bed. I may not even have to be physically touched to feel really sensual. I just feel like, "Oooooh, it's happening!" Then I just let go and go with the flow. A lot of inhibitions are now gone. I used to have worries when I was having sex,

like "Am I doing it right?" It was usually a
performance issue, but now it isn't. I also
worried if I looked "good enough."

INT: *What do you mean when you say "good enough"?*

LISA: There's a lot of that in our society—all these
subliminal messages. I used to see a beautiful
woman in a magazine and think, "Boy, there's
no way I could ever look like her. I'm sure she's
exciting in bed, and I will never be that
exciting because I don't look like that." Or
when I was about to undress in front of a man,
I'd be worrying that he'd see this cottage-cheese
look on my thighs. But now my attitude is,
So *what* if I have a couple extra pounds. I'm
O.K. and I'm going to enjoy myself.

INT: *What's going on in your mind during sex now?*

LISA: It's an inner feeling now—almost like an inner
massage. I don't know what it is. But whatever
has happened, I feel more easily turned on and
my orgasms last and last. I used to think only this
little part—the clitoris—had to be stimulated
to orgasm. But that's not true for me anymore.
I've discovered so many erogenous zones!

INT: *Have your intimate relationships changed?*

LISA: Yes, that's really interesting. In the
relationship I had before—the one with the
guy who left me when he found out I had cancer—I
felt so dependent on him. I used to sit by the
phone wondering, "When is he going to call?

Is he going to call?" I learned not to feel that
dependency anymore. I told myself, "It's going
to be okay if you're alone." And all of a
sudden, this man entered my life—he's great and
accepts me the way I am. What's even more
important is that I accept *myself* the way I am.
And sex is, like, wildly spontaneous. I'll just
meet him at the door and it's like "Waaahhhh!"

INT: *And how does this compare to the way you were
before?*

LISA: Before, it was, like, programmed. It was like
"Let's have a drink first. Let's sit down. How did
your day go?" Then maybe if the mood was all
just right, sex might happen. Now, I notice
when I'm in the mood and I tell him. If he
says, "No, not right now," that's O.K. and I'll say,
"I'm going to bed. If you want to join me, come
join me. Because I'm not letting this good
feeling go!" If he won't join me, I'll go to bed
alone and masturbate. [Laughs joyously.]

INT: *What are your peak sexual times like now?*

LISA: I'm really just tuned in a lot more to myself.
I follow the pleasure, I guess. Like I feel this
nice "trickly" feeling. It's a little warm sensation
that starts in my groin area and touches my belly
button and gives me this little *twing* feeling.
It's a little like a string is being pulled from
my tummy, and I know that as soon as he enters
it's *bam!* and I can become lost in the moment.
It doesn't happen every single time. But
sometimes, just as soon as he enters, I come.

And it's a wonderful body experience—a whole-
body experience. It's really intense.

INT: *Where do you put your focus—your attention—
throughout all this?*

LISA: Actually, nowhere. I don't think about work.
I don't think about my clients. I don't think
about the way I look. I'm just there. I'm just enjoying
the moment. I remember when I used to make
love, I used to think, "Well, I wonder what he
does all day?" I used such thoughts to get
through it. But now I feel like I'm finally part of
the lovemaking. Brad has helped me a lot to not
feel so scared. When I first met him, I was a
little afraid of what he'd think about me because
I'd had a double mastectomy. But then I thought,
"Well, if he can't accept me as I am, that's *his*
problem." So I just let go of that thought. I just
tore off my blouse and said, "This is me. This
is Lisa." And you know what he said? He said,
"You're beautiful." I admit my breasts aren't as
sensual as they once were. Since having the
breast reconstruction surgery, I don't have the
nipple sensations anymore and I used to be very
stimulated by someone just touching my nipples.
But I've transferred my feelings more to other
parts of my body. My doctor, who was very
kind trying to warn me, said, "Lisa, I'm afraid you
may not have the same sexual feelings you once
did." And I told him, "Doctor, I have more
feelings than I know what to do with!"

INT: *You say you masturbate—how does that compare
to sex with a partner?*

Lisa: I do masturbate, but it's not the same as when we're making love; masturbation is more of a quickie. It *does* turn me on when he's there watching me, though.

Int: *Tell me what you see or hear while you're making love.*

Lisa: A lot of times I have music playing. I love soft classical music. But, you know, it's real interesting. When we're making love, I don't hear the music. It's there, but it's sucked right into me and I'm able to hear it inside out. It's hard to explain, but I don't hear my music. It's such a different feeling now. I want to explore, to discover. I want to see and feel everything my body can do. And music contributes to that free-flowing feeling. I also love candlelight. It's so romantic. I have come to realize sensuality is really important.

Int: *What do you focus on during penetration?*

Lisa: Now when he penetrates, I focus on him being inside me, and I feel the walls of my vagina, and I feel the contractions and it stimulates my whole being. It's not just one area anymore.

Int: *Tell me, if you can, how you felt about your mastectomy.*

Lisa: Oh, at first I was livid. But when I got cancer I stopped trying to please everyone else at my expense. Now, I take care of myself. My rage is much less intense. Of course, I get upset and

frustrated at times, but I don't have that rage.
I also think I make better decisions now. I'm more
open to my creativity: ideas flow more easily. I'm
not so overbearing and controlling during
conversations anymore, either. When I'm
talking to someone, I'm really *listening*. When
I talk to you, I want to know about you, what
you feel. I want to understand what's
happening to you and slowly let you discover
me.

INT: *And you say that all of this change began to emerge
when the doctor said you were a miracle?*

LISA: I think that's when it began. I really went
through a major shift in my thinking. Two days
earlier I'd been looking at death row. I was
wondering, "Gosh, should I get my funeral
together?" You know, I was thinking I didn't
want to be a burden on my mom and dad, because
my dad's got cancer, too. It was like I wanted
to take care of the rest of my life so nobody
else would have to. But at the same time I
was fighting. It was like I had two people inside
of me, one of them getting ready to die and the
other one saying, "Just stand back and watch.
There's no way I'm dying. I'm going to fool
you all." I had a battle going on, and the stronger
voice won. Two days after my surgery, I thought,
"To hell with all of you who said I was going
to die. I'm going for it! I'm going to live each
day as fully as I can." And I felt a new perspective
come over me with that decision—like I was
celebrating my rebirth. And now, after two

years, my doctors say there's not a cancer cell
to be found!

INT: *What else is important to you now?*

LISA: Solitude is more important than it's ever been.
I love walking along the ocean and listening to
the waves. I do a lot of reflective thought. I
went through a real humbling experience. I
feel a real inner peace, like the peace a lot of
people say they have when they meet with God.
I don't know what's happened to me, it's hard
to put into words. But it's a nice sensation
from my fingers to my toes. It happens, too, when
I make love. A door has opened and somebody
has shown me a whole new path. Another
change is knowing I can't buy happiness. If
I have the money and see something I want, I'll
buy it. But if I can't afford it, it's okay. Before
I was always trying to keep up with the
Joneses. But now I don't want to *have,* I want
to *feel.* I do have bad moments, of course. Right
before PMS time, I cry. But I've also discovered
my "inner child." I don't mean to sound trite,
but in some ways, I'm like a kid going through
the curiosity stage again. For example, I used
to love the roller coaster and I just thought the
other day, "What fear developed in me that
made me decide I couldn't ride the roller
coaster anymore?" So I'm going to ride the roller
coaster again. I'm going to do that with a lot of
things in my life.

INT: *What about your fantasies—are you enjoying
them more?*

LISA: Oh, yeah. I've even fantasized to orgasm. During those times, I'm not thinking about people having sex or anything like that. I'm just feeling happy. I find it fascinating that I can spark an orgasm with my mind, without any toys or physical touching at all. I'm still learning. I'm just so excited. I want to feel life to the max.

How is it that pain, or a life-threatening experience, sometimes accompanies a sudden supersexual transformation? Because it wakes us up. In the words of C. S. Lewis, "Pain [is] God's megaphone." It's easy to float along through life half-awake when everything's running smoothly. But when faced with a challenge of this magnitude we quickly learn what's important. We start paying attention to what we truly value. And when we do, we awaken to all of life—including the joy of supersex. For Lisa, her breast cancer helped her recognize that all challenges offer opportunities for new depths of understanding. This, of course, does not mean we all have to develop cancer or have a near-death experience before we can awaken to life and achieve our full sexual potential. It only means that somehow we have to seize the challenges presented.

Balance and Harmony—The Wisdom Within

How does it feel when you're in touch with the balance and harmony in your life? How do you live? What do you pay attention to? A few of the people we interviewed exemplify a sense of balance, harmony, and connectedness in their lives that opens them to a kind of "inner wisdom," a reservoir of advice and direction. They seemed to us to be in tune with their internal rhythms, to keep step with their intuition, and to flow with ease along the continuum of controlling and letting go.

Felicia, forty-seven, is one woman who has achieved this joyous level of wisdom. Once an Olympic diver, she now works as an interpreter for the deaf. She wears no makeup and exudes a kind of self-confidence that says, "Here I am, what you see is what you get." When you first meet her, she has a reserved, almost frosty quality that seems intimidating. She has such a direct, honest gaze it's almost as if she has X-ray vision and can look right through you. Once you start talking to her, however, she opens up and engages easily.

Felicia's awakening came in her late twenties, several years after a brutal rape. She recalls, "That was a very bitter, frightening experience because I thought I was going to die. Yet, strangely, it didn't affect my ability to enjoy sex. I think that's because I realized even at the time it was happening that it wasn't a sexual act, but an act of murderous aggression. For about two years after that, I struggled with feelings of depression and even thought of ending my life. I literally had to fight my way back to life and wanting to live. In a way, the rape was a catalyst to help me reexamine my life's purpose. To ask, 'What is it about life that makes me want to hang on?' I spent many nights praying." She also sought meaning by studying the teachings of a great many religious teachers, psychologists, and philosophers—from Jesus, the Buddha, and Martin Buber, to Jung.

Felicia's revelation came during one especially vivid supersexual experience, when she recalls, "I literally became the ocean. I didn't just hear the waves or taste the salt: I *was* the ocean. It absolutely took me by surprise. I don't know how to explain it except to say that I think I moved into another state of consciousness. I have no idea how long it lasted. But this was a mind-body-spirit feeling.

It wasn't just an orgasm. It was beyond orgasm. I became the ocean, then I came back into my body." Felicia's experience had a profound effect in that it gave her a reason for living. "Since that time I have always felt a real spirituality and sacredness in sexuality," she says. "I guess I'd have to say becoming the ocean was the opening that put me in touch with the oneness of all, the idea that I and the universe are one."

Today, Felicia no longer spends much time reading books in search of meaning. She says, "I'm much more into myself nowadays, just living. You know, living for the moment. After years of tearing after the answers, I'm content just to be." Her thoughts as described echo those of the college professor in Chapter 5 who said, "I no longer felt I had to *search* for the meaning because I had *experienced* the meaning."

Despite a hectic schedule, Felicia tries to set aside some time every day to sit in solitude. "I love my mornings," she says. "I like spending an hour or so alone every day before I go to work. I don't always get it. But the inner world is very alive to me, and I like being with it." What does she do during this time? "I just *feel.* Often I'll sip a cup of tea and just let my mind wander until it settles very comfortably on an idea or an image. Or since arranging flowers is a passion of mine, I may just sit and contemplate one of my flower arrangements. I can sit for an hour, just staring at the vase with the rose—just pursuing it sensually. This gives me great pleasure, peace, and a sense of my connection with nature and all living things."

Even though she lives simply, Felicia insists she needs nothing more in her life to be happy. "I own a car and a couple of degrees, but I don't aspire to things very much. I do aspire to land. I want my own little property because I want a garden. I want the security of that. But I have no urge to possess or go after more toys."

What does she most value? "Integration and whole-ness." Asked to elaborate, she explains, "I'm personally trying to pursue the truth of life and how to live it. I'm interested in how to live gracefully, creatively, and in a sense completely. I want to get to the essence of things, whether it be in psychology, philosophy, religion, another person, or a relationship. I want to get down to it."

Getting down to it. Attempting to understand one's essence. This seems to be the overriding goal of most of the people who are reaching toward their full sexual potential, whether they've adopted a lifestyle of simplicity like Felicia, or have ambitions that include greater wealth and influence like others in our study.

Natalie came to a similar realization one night on a winding back road in New England:

I was twenty years old and driving along one night when I rounded a curve and saw a car headed straight toward me on my side of the road. I thought it was a drunk driver. And all I could think of at that moment was, "I cannot die. My room is a mess, and my mother will find my diaphragm!" I was just saying over and over to myself, "I can't die, I can't die. I can't believe this. What's my boyfriend going to do? Oh, man! I just can't die." Then all of a sudden, at the moment my car hydroplaned and flipped over, I felt like my whole body was filled with warm honey. There was a "presence" in the car; that's the only way I can explain it. Sometimes I say that God was there and people look at me like I'm crazy. I didn't see anybody—not a him or a her—but I did feel a presence that was with me. And then all of a sudden I got the idea that what is *is* and what isn't *isn't* and that each day is just right, just the way it should be and that all the days are interconnected, but that every moment is also complete in itself. I know it sounds weird because the accident was a very negative thing to have happened. But it was actually the best experience of my life.

Luckily, I was not hurt. But the next day everything was just very intense: colors were brighter, sounds were keener, everything just seemed more *real*. I didn't change my life in any dramatic way. I didn't change my job or anything. However, the experience made me realize it's better to be *inwardly mobile* than outwardly, upwardly mobile.

Natalie, who became supersexual shortly after this experience, puts in long hours five days a week as an auditor to earn a comfortable living. But, for her, the deepest pleasures in her life come from within and cannot be purchased.

Geena, on the other hand, is a fifty-two-year-old supersexual woman married to a successful corporate attorney. They live in a gracious home and enjoy many of the material comforts of life. The point is not that supersexual women lack possessions or deny themselves material comforts, but that they've come to the realization that what they own and how much they achieve in the world matters far less than who they are.

The Patience to Let Supersex Unfold

Patience is another virtue supersexual women seem to have somehow acquired in our hurried world. Whether they're waiting for an answer to their problems or transcending time and space in a lover's arms, their philosophy seems to be: Try, but don't strain. Asked why she thought patience was so important both in lovemaking and in life, one woman replied, "Have you read *Zorba the Greek?* There's a passage in that novel about a butterfly that says it all."

Looking up the passage, we found the following story. The character whom novelist Nikos Kazantzakis calls

"Boss" has discovered a cocoon in the bark of a tree one morning, just as the butterfly is making a hole in its case and is about to come out. Kazantzakis writes:

> I waited a while, but it was too long appearing and I was impatient. I bent over it and breathed on it to warm it. I warmed it as quickly as I could and the miracle began to happen before my eyes, faster than life. The case opened, the butterfly started slowly crawling out and I shall never forget my horror when I saw how its wings were folded back and crumpled; the wretched butterfly tried with its whole trembling body to unfold them. Bending over it, I tried to help it with my breath. In vain. It needed to be hatched out patiently and the unfolding of the wings should be a gradual process in the sun. Now it was too late. My breath had forced the butterfly to appear all crumpled, before its time. It struggled desperately and, a few seconds later, died in the palm of my hand.
>
> That little body is, I do believe, the greatest weight I have on my conscience. For I realize today that it is a mortal sin to violate the great laws of nature. We should not hurry, we should not be impatient, but we should confidently obey the eternal rhythms.

Supersexual women have learned to trust the rhythms of life, to let everything—including supersex—unfold in its own time. They have learned that they don't have to control everything in their lives to achieve sexual bliss or to be joyous. On the contrary, joy comes to us only when we take responsibility for our lives just to that point where we must let go.

How can you begin finding such balance and sexual richness in your own life? As we've repeatedly said, you already contain this power within you. In many ways, supersex is the natural way to make love—the way we'd all be enjoying sex if we could become fully open to the joys of life. Let's now examine how open you are to pleasure and how you can use a knowledge of your own absorption style to move farther along your supersexual path.

∽ CHAPTER 11 ∾

Finding Your Absorption Style

"When you take a flower in your hand and really look at it," she said, cupping her hand and holding it close to her face, *"it's your world for the moment."*

—Georgia O'Keeffe,
1946 interview in the *New York Post*

The pathway to supersex does not consist of following some lockstep model that guarantees sexual ecstasy. However, there are guidelines to help you on your own personal path to discovery. These include:

- Becoming familiar with your own absorption style
- Noticing your "blocks" to supersexual pleasure
- Making choices to deepen your pleasure

This chapter will show you how to more fully recognize your potential for sexual joy. All you need to begin is an interest in taking the journey.

You know that your ability to enjoy sex, food, a movie, or anything else depends on how open you are to the experience. On the purely physical level, you can't enjoy any sensory experience unless you open your body, your mouth, your eyes, and ears. The psychological openness to, and capacity to immerse oneself in experience, which we have called absorption, is only one aspect of personality. But it is a critical aspect of enjoying supersexual pleasure. Although we are all born with a certain tendency to be a "low" or "high" absorber, this is not a fixed part of our personality. It is merely a capacity or potential that is shaped and modified by daily experiences.

But why is absorption so important? Because it reflects the way you think and the attentional choices you make—what you focus on. Whether you tend to be high, medium, or low in absorption reflects what you notice, how you notice it (what senses you use and how deeply they are involved), whether you find something to be pleasurable or not, or whether you disregard the event or situation entirely. Consider this example: Florence's partner leaves an unexpected bouquet of roses for her on the kitchen table with a note that reads, "Just because." A low absorber might tend to initially wonder "What's the real occasion?" or "How could he afford those flowers on our limited budget?" While these are reasonable questions, the beauty or fragrance of the roses might only be experienced secondarily—or not at all. If the concern about budget or motivation is primary, it may overshadow the potential for sensory enjoyment. A high absorber might respond to the event differently—taking time to first smell the roses or rearrange them artfully in a vase while admiring their beauty. She might extend the enjoyment by pausing during the day to recall their fragrance or to re-create their visual attractiveness in her mind. Questions may occur as well, but the high absorber will release these and refocus on pleasure. Long after the roses have faded, a high absorber will continue to enjoy them through the richness and vividness of her recollections.

Low absorbers tend to be more functional in their approach to situations and solutions while high absorbers tend to be more imaginative. These are clearly generalizations, and the responses of most high or low absorbers can not be uniformly categorized as either "imaginative" or "functional." There is a spectrum of absorption with many levels and combinations. It's important to understand that high absorbers are not emotionally healthier than low absorbers. There are strengths and limitations to each attentional style, and both are necessary to wholeness. Although it is true that it is the high absorbers who become deeply "lost" in supersex, it is important to recognize that each style has its own appropriate function. In an extreme case, if a high absorber consistently experiences events from the perspective of her own internal reality, she may become so self-consumed that she detaches from external events in a way that goes beyond the boundaries of conventional behavior. She becomes extremely self-absorbed. Conversely, the consistent low absorber can become exclusively preoccupied with tasks—"functions"—to the detriment of her imaginative self, and what she loves and feels. Both extremes result in imbalance. What is necessary to access optimum joy, sexually as in all other aspects of life, is to develop a flexibility in your focus of attention, not to become trapped at either end of the absorption continuum, and to be able to flow back and forth freely between functionality and imagination, reason and emotion, holding on and letting go, impulse and control, as one chooses. Key ingredients shared by women who enjoy supersex are flexibility, balance, and the ability to access pleasure in many forms.

By using the same absorption tool as we initially used to screen our subjects, you will learn how deeply absorbed you're presently able to be. You can then discover how your focus may be restricting your pleasure and learn to recognize opportunities to enhance your sexual enjoyment. If you discover that your present style limits your sexual pleasure, then it may be time for some change—to expand your options. The choice will be yours.

Before reading further, find a pen or pencil and take a few minutes to respond to the statements below. Remember that there are no right or wrong answers. Although by now you can probably guess how the women in our study answered, read each question and respond quickly without much deliberation—your first response is the one to enter. If, while taking this quiz, you find yourself wishing you could agree with more statements, that's an important message to notice—it may be a signal that you are interested in learning more about your potential for supersex. Simply mark each statement as True or False.

1. Sometimes I feel and experience things as I did when I was a child.

2. I can be greatly moved by eloquent or poetic language.

3. While watching a movie, TV show, or play, I may become so involved that I forget about myself and my surroundings and experience the story as if it were real and I were actually taking part in it.

4. If I stare at a picture and then look away from it, I can sometimes "see" an image of the picture, almost as if I were still looking at it.

5. Sometimes I feel as if my mind could envelop the whole world.

6. I like to watch cloud shapes and changes in the sky.

7. If I wish, I can imagine (or daydream) some things so vividly that they hold my attention as a good movie or story does.

8. I think I really know what some people mean when they talk about mystical experiences.

9. I sometimes "step outside" my usual self and experience an entirely different state of being.

10. Textures such as wool, sand, or wood sometimes remind me of colors or music.

11. Sometimes I experience things as if they were doubly real.

12. When I listen to music, I can get so caught up in it that I don't notice anything else.

13. If I wish, I can imagine that my body is so heavy that I could not move if I wanted to.

14. I can somehow sense the presence of another person before I actually see or hear him or her.

15. The crackling flames of a wood fire stimulate my imagination.

16. It is sometimes possible for me to be completely immersed in nature or in art and feel as if my whole state of consciousness has somehow been temporarily altered.

17. Different colors have distinctive and special meanings for me.

18. I am able to wander off into my own thoughts while doing a routine task and actually forget that I am doing the task, and then find a few minutes later that I have completed it.

19. I can sometimes recollect certain past experiences in my life with such clarity and vividness that it is like, or almost like, reliving them again.

20. Things that might seem meaningless to others often make sense to me.

21. While acting in a play, I think I can really feel the emotions of the character and "become" her or him for the time being, forgetting both myself and the audience.

22. My thoughts often don't occur as words, but as visual images.

23. I often take delight in small things (like the five-pointed star shape that appears when you cut an apple across the core, or the colors in soap bubbles).

24. When listening to organ music or other powerful music, I sometimes feel as if I am being lifted into the air.

25. Sometimes I can change noise into music by the way I listen to it.

26. Some of my most vivid memories are called up by scents and smells.

27. Certain pieces of music remind me of pictures of moving patterns of color.

28. I often know what someone is going to say before he or she says it.

29. I often have "physical memories," for example, after I've been swimming I may still feel as if I'm in the water.

30. The sound of a voice can be so fascinating to me that I can just go on listening to it.

31. At times I somehow feel the presence of someone who is not physically there.

32. Sometimes thoughts and images come to me without the slightest effort on my part.

33. I find that different odors have different colors.

34. I can be deeply moved by a sunset.

Now add up the number of true statements. This scale was intended to be taken as part of a 300-item personality inventory and it is not scientifically valid when taken out of context. Therefore, your score will no doubt be higher now than it would have been in the context of the entire inventory. However, it can give you some idea of how far you have come on your supersexual journey and will offer clues as to which strategies you can try if you'd like to go further. There are no certainties or absolutes here. But our research suggests that if you scored somewhere between 0 and 14, you are probably a low absorber; a score of 15 to 21 suggests you are a medium absorber; and if you're a 22 or above, you may well be a high absorber like the women in our study who describe supersex. The higher your score, the more you are presently able to immerse yourself in whatever you love—including sexual ecstasy.

Discovering Your Absorption Clusters

What else can you learn about yourself from taking this quiz? You can learn not only how high of an absorber you are but also what kind of absorber, including whether you pay attention to engaging "external" events (like poetic language) or respond to spontaneously generated "internal" imaginings. The thirty-four items of the absorption scale fall into seven "clusters" which describe varying components of absorption. These clusters have been adapted from Tellegen and we have applied them to supersexual absorption.* Each cluster is a measure of what you are doing now and what has already proven to be useful in your experience of pleasure. By identifying your key areas for absorption, you will be ready to use them to build your "connection" to ecstasy as described in Chapter 13.

So return to your absorption quiz and write down the numbers of the items you marked True. Then locate the item under its cluster. Read the description of each cluster to see if it is consistent with how you experience yourself. Remember that these are descriptions of your current style of absorption, and indicate current areas of strength.

*For technical note on the Absorption Scale, see Author's note p. 239

Cluster 1: Focusing on images and tuning out distractions
(Questions 3, 7, 12, 21)

If you have marked True to questions in Cluster 1, you may focus on things so vividly and completely that you block out distractions in the environment. When you are making love with your partner, you may not hear the telephone ringing or the dog scratching on the door. You become so focused on what you enjoy that you may become lost in a moment of pleasure.

If you would like to go deeper in Cluster 1, consider trying the following: During sex, keep your focus on what you enjoy. Pay attention when your mind wanders away from the pleasure and gently redirect your focus. By paying attention to the pleasurable images, feelings, or sensations, the distractions will fade into the background. The more often you do this, the more natural it will become.

Cluster 2: Responding to engaging "external" cues
(Questions 2, 6, 15, 23, 30, 34)

If you have responded True to questions in Cluster 2, you feel emotional stirrings in response to engaging external cues, situations, or events. A romantic card or a message on your office voice mail from your lover may bring a warm glow; your partner's fragrance may be sexually exciting; you may be sensitive to sensations—the feel of skin touching skin, pleasant smells, tastes, sounds. When enjoying pleasure (if you are on the high end of this cluster) you can stay focused on the sensation and may begin to drift beyond the physical experience (see Cluster 3). If you are on the lower end of this cluster (with fewer True responses to these questions), you may stay focused on the sensation itself without moving to a change in conscious awareness. You may describe your orgasms as "satisfying" or "a wonderful release" and you may keep your attention focused on the good feeling in your genitals, breasts, or other areas of your body. Depending on your precise level of absorption, or depth of focus, you may or may not drift in your attention or find yourself distracted.

To enhance or deepen your absorption in Cluster 2, take time to linger on emotional stirrings you feel, allowing them to deepen. Experiment with intensifying your enjoyment of senses by approaching each joyful moment from a fresh perspective. For example, if you've received a flower and would ordinarily simply smell it, intentionally notice other sensory aspects of the flower. Look at it, feel the softness of the petals against your cheek or your fingertips (notice the difference), place it in different light and admire the subtle or not so subtle changes. Consider the meaning of the gift and notice your response to receiving it. If you feel happy, surprised, proud, or even sad—feel it deeply inside of yourself. Just noticing or paying attention to your feelings will heighten the feeling for you. You can deepen your sensory enjoyment of sexual feelings/pleasures in the same way. (See also the section "Suspending Certainty and Cultivating a Beginner's Mind" on p. 196.)

Cluster 3: Deeply
responding to engaging "external" cues leading to alterations in conscious awareness
(Questions 16, 18, 24)

Cluster 3 is a deepening of Cluster 2. If you have responded to questions in Cluster 3, you tend to experience deeply intense emotional stirrings in response to cues, situations, or events, and allow yourself to flow with the pleasure. You may begin your passion by focusing your attention on an "external" event (studying your partner's eyes, or an erotic touch) and then allow yourself to enter the experience so deeply that you may feel swept away or taken to a different dimension. As if you have given up on the idea of containing the feeling—or holding on to it—you let go and permit the pleasure to steer you to your next level of passion.

To enhance or deepen your experience in Cluster 3, begin again with a sensation that captures your attention and stirs your emotions. Allow yourself to focus as completely as possible on that experience. Are you aware of stopping yourself at some "boundary" where the enjoyment "ends"? There is no boundary to enjoyment because the potential for pleasure is limitless. When you have created a safe environment for yourself, you will allow yourself to relax deeply into the pleasure and allow it to take you to new dimensions of discovery. Experiment with sensual pleasure and see what might "stop" you from letting go. Perhaps you have concerns, worries, or pressures that need to be addressed. Recognizing these "blocks" may be all that is needed to grow to another level of consciousness—a level that can go beyond pleasure to infinite joy. (See also the section, "Trusting Your Partner and Yourself," on page 190.)

Cluster 4: Vividly re-experiencing the past
(Questions 1, 4, 19)

If you have responded True to questions in Cluster 4, you are able to recall past events with vividness and clarity. You may be able to hear your wedding music many years later, feel the touch of your lover in his or her absence, or enjoy the memories of passionate sexual moments again and again. You may be able to have high sexual arousal or orgasm through your recollections of past events alone. You may also be able to transform sensations by "seeing," in your mind's eye, a snapshot of the first time you and your lover kissed and recapture the heat of that time years later. Or you may listen to your partner's breathing or heartbeat and connect it (in your mind or consciousness) to the rhythmic contractions of orgasm.

To deepen your experience of Cluster 4, you can experiment with a variety of ways to access past events and feelings. You can reread old love letters, poems, or valentines you wrote or received. Play old records, read your diary, smell your or your partner's favorite scents; look at a photo album of your wedding day or a special trip—and allow yourself to gently drift along with the sensations and notice whatever images emerge. See how clearly you can visualize that image and stay with it until it changes. See how it changes. Don't be critical of anything that emerges. Some of the events may be tinged with sadness. The more vividly you can imagine past events, the more directly you will learn about your full range of passion.

Cluster 5: Daydreaming and fantasy
(Questions 22, 32)

If you have responded True to questions in Cluster 5, you can easily become lost in daydreams or the enjoyment of sexual fantasy—from a fleeting image to a full-length "movie" that unfolds in your mind. You find yourself easily drifting into pleasurable scenes and letting go of outside distractions. Images seem to come to you with visual clarity in an effortless way. Sexually, you can transport yourself to a favorite setting with your "ideal" lover and enjoy the best your mind can offer. You may find that you have awakened from an especially erotic dream feeling as if you have had a "no hands" orgasm.

To deepen your appreciation of daydreaming, give yourself permission to notice your sexual images whenever they may occur. Instead of letting them rush by almost unnoticed, take a moment to savor them or write them down so that you can enjoy them again later. If a fragment of an image should occur, allow it to unfold like a movie. Notice how one image sometimes transforms into another. Don't try to connect the images in any logical way, just follow them as if you are on a great adventure. If no image comes to mind, recall a movie scene or book passage that touched you. (See also the section, "Enhancing Your Enjoyment of Senses, Images, and Fantasies" on page 200.)

Cluster 6: Cross-sensory experience
(Questions 10, 17, 25, 26, 27, 29, 33)

If you have responded True to questions in Cluster 6, you have learned to combine your enjoyment of your senses in non-traditional, creative, and exciting ways. Colors may have special meanings or certain odors may be associated with different colors. Seeing the color blue may remind you of the sweet taste of your lover's mouth when you kissed by the blue-green sea while at Saint Barth's. That certain color can bring it all back to you.

If you would like to deepen your ability to have cross-sensory experiences, you might begin with a box of crayons or paint samples. Allow your mind to scan the spectrum of colors and settle on a hue that attracts you. Explore your attraction by asking yourself what tastes, sights, sounds, or smells this color might evoke. For example, if you are attracted to the color green, perhaps it reminds you of spring grass, the color of your lover's eyes, or the taste of fresh mint. Or perhaps you have an olfactory response to the color and may smell pine needles. Pay particular attention to any unlikely sensory modalities that may just come to you—temperature, texture, brightness, solidity. They may emerge spontaneously. Experiment by starting with a fragrance or a sound. Don't struggle to make anything happen, just notice what does. The more you attend to these possibilities for cross-sensory perception, the more they will become part of your absorption spectrum. (See also the section on "Enhancing Your Enjoyment of Senses, Images, and Fantasies" on page 200.)

Cluster 7: Spiritual connection
(Questions 5, 8, 9, 11, 14, 20, 28, 31)

If you have responded True to questions in Cluster 7, you have a special sensitivity to spirituality and may feel an *I-Thou* connection with your partner. You have an enhanced focus of awareness and way of thinking that allows you to transcend physical boundaries to access another realm of experience—beyond what can rationally be defined. Women who are highly developed in their spiritual connections may feel a oneness or harmony with the universe through nature, their work, and their sexuality. They often describe the "connection of auras," the "blending of souls" or the "synchronicity of heartbeats" while making love.

If you are interested in deepening your spiritual connection, it is important that you notice where and when you feel this dimension in your life. Is it associated with a particular place, person, or state of mind? Practice placing yourself there physically or mentally, quiet your mind using any approach that works for you, and open it to whatever experience is offered to you. This is one of the more challenging dimensions of absorption to "prescribe" yet the ingredients are quite simple: creating a safe environment, trusting your own inner wisdom, and acknowledging the power of a spiritual potential that comes from you and through you. In reading the descriptions of these clusters, keep in mind that they are not arranged in a linear or sequential manner (with the exception of Clusters 2 and 3). All of these clusters were grouped together based on the information we obtained from the women having supersex and the experiences they reported to us. Supersexual women have the ability to access most of, if not all, the clusters. But even those women can go further because each cluster has infinite potential. You may have had some of the experiences to a small degree on one occasion or have had many of the experiences frequently. The more clusters you can endorse and the deeper you go within each grouping, the more likely you are to experience supersex.

Look at the following diagram. It illustrates the multidimensional nature of the absorption spectrum. Notice there are three directions for enhancement of absorption.

Absorption Spectrum

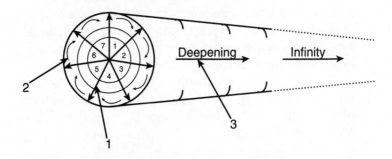

1. Each cluster can be **individually expanded**, e.g., you can **add** senses that you enjoy or vary your images/fantasies.
2. You can **add** clusters.
3. You can **deepen** each/all clusters to infinity.

So you are now much more aware of what kind of absorber you are currently. If you are on the low or medium end of the absorption spectrum, you may notice that your items from the absorption quiz fall under Cluster 2. Low absorbers tend to have an external focus which can naturally deepen (as described in Cluster 3). Wherever you may be on your journey, you have already started to go further. Becoming aware of your place on the absorption continuum will free you to notice options or alternatives that may have passed by unnoticed before now.

Let's now meet several women at various points on the absorption spectrum. As you read these case histories, think about the ways you would like to develop your own pleasure. Perhaps you will be able to identify with aspects of these interviews. Following the cases we have provided questions you can consider to enrich your absorption.

Pearl is a woman who is a low absorber—scoring 11 on the absorption scale. She is a clear-thinking, straight-talking sixty-three-year-old mathematics teacher who has been married for forty-two years—but many of those years have been unsatisfying ones. She reports not having had "partner sex" for the past eight years, but being very satisfied with masturbation, and that she is now "working" on leaving her husband, Ralph: "We're just two very different people," she says. "But the timing has had to be right for me to leave."

At the start of the interview, when asked to describe an experience when she was "lost in the moment" she replied, "I'm not one of those artsy-fartsy people, you know, one of those people that gets lost in a moment. . . . I'm really a technical person and a realist—no fantasies for me."

This condensed session gives an example of a woman who feels confident in her decisions about her own sexuality and has chosen, for now, not to go further.

PEARL: But . . . there was this one time [a twinkle in her eye] when I heard bells—would you like to hear about that?

INT: *Tell me about it as clearly as you can remember it.*

PEARL: Ralph and I were dating—oh, God—forty-two years ago. It was after we had gone swimming. We had this little pond on my family's farm and we swam across to this point and then, [she breaks into a smile] we had fun on the other side! [laughs heartily] We were both twenty or twenty-one and it was very exhilarating swimming to the point. And of course we'd be alone. It was a very warm, intimate time. We didn't have sex—intercourse, I mean—but we did a lot of kissing. Once, after we'd been swimming and he was walking me home—well, I heard bells ring when he kissed me.

INT: *Do you remember where you were at the time?*

PEARL: Yes, yes, we were in the front hall of the apartment building he lived in. You know, I used to hear this in the movies, that bells would ring. I didn't know it really happened. But it did happen to me—that one time.

INT: *How about during other sexual moments?*

PEARL: Oh, I remember many times that I would say were exciting. When we were young it was the making out in the car routine. It wasn't like they do nowadays, going to a motel or anything like that. It was always a car situation, after a dance or something.

INT: *You say many times were exciting. Can you describe how and where you would feel this excitement?*

PEARL: Well, I had orgasms—and I felt them in my body, where else? Look, I'm not a very imaginative or creative person and I like it that way. I have both of my feet planted on the ground and my head is not in the clouds. But I've had great sex in my many years. I can remember somebody—when I wasn't doing well with Ralph—telling me, "You ought to have an affair." They were trying to tell me that because I hadn't had sex with anyone else. And I would say, "I don't know." And they said, "You really don't know what good sex is because you've only been with one man." And I said, "Well, how can you do any better than this: that when you both get done, both of your bodies feel like satin?" That person never said another word to me again!

INT: *So during the best times you remember feeling like satin?*

PEARL: I never had any problems with sex—my body got aroused easily and I liked the feeling of release.

INT: *Did you ever forget about your surroundings during those "satin" moments?*

PEARL: No ... I never drifted off, I knew exactly what I was doing. As I say, I am not a fantasy person. [she says this with a kind of pride] I stay in reality and the reality is great for me.

INT: *How about when you masturbate—do you fantasize
then?*

PEARL: [long, thoughtful pause] No. Masturbation
is a wonderful physical release for me. It's just
a tension that builds up and a way to relieve
that and feel relaxed. Of course I know I could
learn how to use my imagination more—because
if sex felt like satin that was a kind of fantasy—but
I don't choose to. I like the feeling of being
very present, if you know what I mean. I'm
kind of a "nuts and bolts" person. Maybe that's
why I like mathematics so much—fitting the pieces
together in some logical way.

INT: *Can you tell me about your relationship with
Ralph?*

PEARL: He's a real dreamer. I remember that we had
a wonderful sexual life and for me there was
nothing missing—no matter what was wrong
with us, we had good sex. Then we went through
a lot of trauma, raising the kids in the sixties,
and he lost his job. Twenty years ago, he just
lost everything and pulled away from me
completely. Maybe he needed to blame me. He
doesn't feel he's adequate and now, after all of
these years, I don't feel he's adequate either.

INT: *Where does that leave you?*

PEARL: It leaves me with the reality that we had some
very good times, but they came to an end some
time ago. The hardest part was giving up the
one dream I had for our relationship. Ralph

and I—we did a lot of traveling when we were
first married—would see this wonderful
couple in their seventies. The woman would be
standing tall and straight and the man would be
bent over his cane a bit. And there would be
an aura about them. And I'd say to Ralph,
"See, that's what I want you and I to be." And
he said that would never be because I killed off
his dreams. And I felt that he killed off mine.
He just felt that he had become a loser in his
life and tried to blame me—but I decided to not
take that responsibility. But I really feel O.K. about
myself because I have my own strength and
profession—Lord knows I have worked hard
for it. People sometimes think you have to have
a man to survive, especially from my generation,
but it's not so.

INT: *What about the dream you held so dearly?*

PEARL: It was just that—a dream. Sure it would have
been nice, but not all nice things come to pass.
I suppose I've learned to accept that the dream
won't be. You need to understand that I'm a
mathematician—a scientist. I definitely don't read
a novel unless it's a historical novel or some
informational book on nutrition or something
else. I was having a real hard time living with
this man, and I was questioning myself for years.
I'm happy with life and I'm finally ready to leave
him. I don't need his dependency anymore.
I don't think I ever did.

INT: *And sexually?*

PEARL: [she smiles] I have a great time masturbating in my "down-to-earth way" and I feel very content.

Pearl is an example of a low absorber who chooses and prefers to stay grounded in reality. Although there is some lingering regret and resentment, she is working to resolve those feelings in therapy. She continues to feel healthy and productive on her job, has many friends, and spends many loving moments with her grandchildren. About eight months after this interview, we happened to meet and she informed me (with a very relieved look) that she had found the strength to divorce Ralph and reported doing very well.

Questions to Ponder If You're a Low Absorber:

If you're a low absorber and want to move farther along the road to supersex, here are some questions to consider:

- Where do you think you learned to think of yourself as a "practical" or "realistic" kind of person? Where did you learn what to "realistically" expect from sexuality? Was sexual pleasure part of your expectation?
- Do you think that your "realistic" perspective has limited you?
- Recall a time when you felt creative, spontaneous, or imaginative. A time, perhaps, when sex was unplanned. How did that moment get started? Would you like to feel those moments more often?
- What brings you joy? What are your favorite sensory experiences? Think back to a moment of high enjoyment. Did you have to be in a particular "frame of

mind"? How did it begin? How were you feeling about yourself at the time? Did your relationship have anything to do with it? In what way?

- How long has it been since you have done something "fun" for yourself (gotten a massage, soaked in a tub, gone to the art museum, bought yourself something "frivolous")?

A Triad of Medium Absorbers

The next three women have gone farther along the supersexual path. Marlene (who scored 15 on the absorption scale), Cassandra (who scored 17), and Colleen (who scored 20) share something of the same challenge: each has had to reconsider her belief that some aspect of herself or her life must be perfect before she can let go and be happy.

Marlene, a forty-four-year-old married stockbroker, came into therapy because critical thoughts about how well she was performing kept her from feeling spontaneous and open with her husband, Tony. As a result, she was often bored with sex and, after lovemaking, felt unfulfilled.

The feeling that she would be criticized if she failed to perform perfectly didn't sweep over her only when she was making love; it was a pattern expressed in many parts of her life. At work, for example, she had once loved her job and worked well with her boss. After a company reorganization, she felt less secure with her new boss and began feeling pressure to perform to please her.

The first step Marlene had to take to move closer to supersex and a more stress-free life was to realize that she was creating this unrealistic expectation to be perfect. Shortly after she recognized this simple fact, she felt more control over her choices and less stress.

For her, the situation in her work life paralleled her sexual problems and brought some new realizations. The following is an excerpt of her description of some changes she is beginning to see on her journey to supersex.

INT: *Marlene, you said that work had been fun. What was the fun part of work for you?*

MARLENE: The fun part was being with people I enjoyed. When they left, and then it wasn't the same group of people, I had a hard time getting used to the new, more critical supervisory feeling at work. What I've learned is that although my supervisors are more critical, I still have choices about how I will interpret and respond to criticism. I need to produce an acceptable level of work, but I don't have to drive myself so hard. I was setting such unreasonable expectations—I was my own worst supervisor. It just resulted in my feeling anxious all of the time and I did less than my best work because of it.

INT: *So you found a way to stop worrying about the real and imagined expectations from your supervisors and from inside of yourself, and started relaxing more. How did you do that?*

MARLENE: For years I've been telling myself to stop worrying, but something over the last months just clicked.

INT: *What was that?*

MARLENE: The discovery that worrying and being
nervous and anxious wouldn't change things.
I learned to step back and to be less critical of
myself and to relax much more. I also have learned
to be less critical of other people—like my
husband and my children.

INT: *How has your making this change—being less critical
of yourself and others—affected you in other ways?
You came to see me originally because you were
unhappy with your level of sexual interest with
Tony.*

MARLENE: I feel more confident and more relaxed
with myself. From our first session I realized
that this is the way I thought I was and had
to be—it never really dawned on me that I'm forty-
four years old and I don't have to be critical of
myself. Sometimes I get anxious and still clam
up with Tony—but I've found a way out of this
and it's come from thinking about how comfortable
I am when I'm playing golf. It's a time when I
don't feel my mind thinking so much and I
just relax naturally into the swing. I just step
up to the ball, don't even think about it—I just
feel good and everything feels right and you don't
think about what you're going to do, you just
do it!

INT: *Where does that feeling and swing come from?
How is it created?*

MARLENE: It comes from inside—someplace. I
know that it's nothing forced because I've tried
to force it and it doesn't work then. It just happens.

INT: *Where do you put your mind when that inner swing happens?*

MARLENE: I'm just right there, focusing everything on the ball and not really noticing anything or anyone else. I think that's why golfing is so relaxing for me. I also know that when I'm playing with someone I'm trying to impress, I can get critical of myself on the golf course, too, and it's all shot.

INT: *So you've noticed that when you're critical of yourself at work or when playing golf, you don't play your best game. How have you learned to shut that critical part off when you play golf?*

MARLENE: I just recognize that I'm getting distracted and put my attention back on the ball and relax. Then I find that my focus comes back.

INT: *Can you think of how this transfers to having sex with Tony? Tell me about that.*

MARLENE: Well, sexually, I've noticed that I've also been critical of myself and that now I have more self-confidence and don't try so hard, so sex has been much more relaxing, more natural, and more spontaneous.

INT: *Give me an example.*

MARLENE: The kids were out of the house two nights ago and I told Tony I wanted to make love. I didn't worry about planning for it or making it perfect, I just let my mind be in the room with Tony and focused on what I was feeling. I wasn't feeling worried or distracted—I was just enjoying him and the feelings I was having. If I had been distracted I would have recognized it, and then let it go by focusing back on the pleasure the way you suggested. I was home alone and I really enjoyed touching him. There were no worries or anxieties and I really focused on the way he felt—the little beard stubble on his face that I love and the clean fresh smell of his skin—I really love the way he smells. In the past, when my thoughts distracted me, I didn't feel as connected to my own feelings and to him. Tony told me that he was so happy that I was pleasing myself and enjoying my time with him. I feel that I'm beginning to get to know the me that is inside and to connect with her—becoming more intimate with myself seems to be the most important step here.

INT: *Absolutely. So at work, while golfing, and with Tony, when you are really there and are not distracted by your worries, you feel much more pleasure and satisfaction. Letting the feelings direct your golf swing and direct your touch.*

MARLENE: Yes—it's great. It's hard to describe the feeling. I just feel so much better and more unburdened. Developing that inner focus has made such a difference. Instead of focusing on outside criticism, I focus on what I like. I had never thought about "What would make me happy?" Instead I thought about "What should be done or what needs to be done?" Thinking about what would make me happy has been a

new idea and has created a difference in how
I experience myself. I only allowed myself pleasure
in a few areas—now I see that doing what I
want to do (from an internal place) brings me
the most happiness. I know it will take some
practice—and I have to pay attention not to try
too hard—it's just so exciting to make these
steps and I want more and more.

Like many low and low-medium absorbers, Marlene is
strongest in Cluster 2. She resonates most intensely to
those pleasures in the outside, "real" world (the clean
fresh smell of her lover's skin, the beard stubble on his
face) rather than the more abstract dimensions within her
(such as vivid memories of the past, spiritual connections,
or daydreams). Looking over Marlene's journey, we see
that to move higher up the absorption scale, she could
choose to deepen her appreciation of those sensations she
already loves (that natural golf swing) and to learn to value
that special part of her consciousness—the effortless, natural part of her being. She also needed to realize that her
struggles for perfection were limiting her joy.

Although Marlene has come to understand her own
blocks to supersex through therapy, many women move
along on their journey to supersex without the assistance
of formal therapy by listening to their own inner guidance,
paying attention to the moments in their lives which bring
them profound happiness, and taking note of how that happiness is blocked in sexual relationships.

Cassandra is a forty-seven-year-old banker who scored
17 on the absorption scale. She has two grown children
and has been divorced from her childhood sweetheart for
five years. She is an attractively dressed woman who takes
pride in her appearance. "When I dress up, I just feel bet-

ter all over," she says cheerfully. But her dark brown eyes fill with tears as she talks about her divorce. "I loved him, but he was an alcoholic, and I know that divorce was the best choice for me. It was just very sad to leave my first love." Cassandra is overweight, and acknowledges that she often "turns to food" to fill her in the absence of love. Although she is aware of a passionate part of herself, she refers to it as the "outrageous bad girl."

She is one of many women in our sample who has difficulty reconciling her passion with her intrinsic "goodness." The following is an excerpt of a follow-up interview designed to help Cassandra identify her unconscious decisions to suppress her passion in order to be a "good" girl. In this session you can see her becoming aware of her choice to rethink this false dichotomy of good vs. bad, and redefine her joyous "self" in less pejorative, more self-affirming ways.

> CASSANDRA: It's interesting that you happened to call today because I was feeling a little low. The man that I'm involved with right now has "walls" that he puts up and I feel closed out. When he puts up his walls, then I put up mine and there's no intimacy. But then there's a part of me that says, "That's his stuff and why are you allowing it to affect you?"

> INT: *So there's a voice inside of you that's advising you?*

> CASSANDRA: Yes. It recognizes that I close down when I don't have to and really prevent myself from enjoying whatever is there to enjoy.

> INT: *So part of you chooses to close down, and part of you recognizes you have other options?*

CASSANDRA: I guess I never thought of it as a choice—
it's how I've always reacted. When someone I care
about closes down, I get afraid of rejection or
something—and I pull away too. It sounds
different hearing you say it's a choice that I make.

INT: *Can you think about how you bring yourself
pleasure—real pleasure?*

CASSANDRA: Well, I like to be outside in nature
and feel most free then. I like listening to the
sounds of nature. At lunch I've started taking
a walk outside with my friends and I love that.
I can let go of my worries when I do that. I
find that I can lift myself out of negativity when
I decide to listen to that voice inside that reminds
me how good it is to be alive. But then there
are times when I close down too.

INT: *When do you "close down"?*

CASSANDRA: I think when I'm with a partner who
closes me out, puts up walls, and I feel like
I'm left out—missing something.

INT: *So when you're with a partner who puts up walls,
you close down. At other times you open up to nature
and open up to your inner voice by saying
something positive to yourself. Is that correct?*

CASSANDRA: It seems that way.

INT: *How do you think that this decision you make
to open up or close down affects you sexually?
If you open up, what might you open up to?*

CASSANDRA: I'm afraid that I would open up to
something that would be outrageous. As I get
older, I think that I say the wrong things or should
screen what I say more. And this outrageous part
is dying to get out! [She laughs loudly.] But
I was taught that only bad girls say what's
really on their mind and good girls are quiet and
think before they speak. There's this handsome
guy at work that is strong and very
attractive—very tall with a little-boy charm—
lives on a farm, but wears a suit to work. This
is very attractive to me. When he drives by where
I take a walk during lunch, he stops his car
and usually talks—yesterday he stopped his
car and I asked him where he'd been the last
week and that I've missed seeing him. His face
got red, and I worried that I had said
something outrageous—after all, good girls
shouldn't be that forward.

INT: *Is that what you believe—that you were too forward
and not a "good" girl?*

CASSANDRA: Well, not really, but there's that part
of me again—that "throw-back" part—that keeps
me in the dark ages. I can't believe that I still
refer to myself as a "girl," after all, I am almost
forty-eight!

INT: *So, you're noticing that you still refer to yourself
as a girl rather than a woman and you're trying
to be "good." Tell me, how do you think good
little girls and bad little girls act?*

CASSANDRA: Let's see . . . good little girls are
quiet, withdrawn, and don't say what they feel
and bad little girls [pauses] say what they feel.

INT: *Which ones have the most fun?*

CASSANDRA: [immediately responds] The bad little
girls [laughs].

INT: *So I think we see that the outrageous, fun part
of you is kept reined in very tightly—and how come?*

CASSANDRA: Because it will be offensive to
someone, I suppose. I'm afraid of offending
people. I worry about the fact that my comments
might upset people. . . . I guess I know how to
have fun.

INT: *Your worry about offending others limits your
fun. But you say you know how to have fun; how
would you do that?*

CASSANDRA: I really have the most fun when I
take a risk and say what I feel and not worry
about the other person's reaction. I have to learn
to not dwell on how what I say affects others—to
pay attention to what makes me the happiest.
I know I'm basically a good person, and would
never intentionally hurt someone, but I suppose
that I worry about that too much. I really stop
my spontaneity.

INT: *What happens when you do decide to shut off
the concerns about the other person; how do you
feel* Inside?

CASSANDRA: I can sometimes shut it off—and I
feel so *Empowered*—and I can do that; I just wish
I could do it more often.

INT: *You say that you "wish"—how could you learn
to do that more often?*

CASSANDRA: All I really need to do, I guess, is notice
all the times I don't do it and then make a
conscious effort to do it—hmmm.

INT: *And then what would happen?*

CASSANDRA: [long pause] I think I would feel more
like the free, happy me—more happy a lot
more often.

INT: *So the choice of having joy is before you. Do you
think that the same choice to stay open and not
shut down is there for you when you have sex?*

CASSANDRA: Definitely, but sometimes the
insecure part of me pulls away—the part that
wants to be a "good girl"—and I use food to fill
me at those times because it seems so much
safer, no risk involved. I can see that I stuff
down so much of my own feelings—my anger,
my sadness, so many things—and I don't easily
let go to feeling the "raw feelings."

INT: *When do you most feel in touch with the raw
feelings, the passion inside you? When do you stop
reining yourself in and let yourself feel some joy?*

CASSANDRA: Mostly with music. When I was driving over here in the car, I had Michael Bolton blasting as loud as you can ever imagine and I was singing along in the car, bopping around. For a second I thought, "What if someone sees me," but I said, "Oh, that's their problem," and just continued. I love music—and I like it loud.

INT: *So music is one way that you do what you like. How do you feel when you listen to your music?*

CASSANDRA: I don't know. It just takes care of everything—the sadness, anger, all the emotions inside that I suppress. Then the real passionate Cassandra emerges! Sometimes I feel like I'm just really gone because nothing else is there, just me and my music.

INT: *And what happens sexually?*

CASSANDRA: Maybe I just stop the passion from coming out. I know I do this sexually because I can feel myself getting excited and getting more and more into the turn-on. Then I begin to notice that maybe he's not so excited, and I begin to wonder if I'm being outrageous or a "bad" girl and I think what I do is just stop myself from going further— *Wow*—how interesting. I really want to act more passionately with this guy, but I've just been afraid of what he'd think of that "bad" part of me!

INT: *You need to think more about this label of "bad girl" or "outrageous" that you have given to your "fun side." Thinking this way has really limited your ability to give yourself pleasure.*

CASSANDRA: I know. I see how I really do a number on myself that way. I really like that part of myself. I only feel really me—really happy— when I let my outrageous part out.

INT: *Could you reconsider this: what if what you've been calling the "bad" girl is really the "good" girl!*

CASSANDRA: [Laughs] That feels so good to think of myself that way. I wouldn't have to be so afraid of involving myself in what I like if I thought about that part of me as good—I wouldn't suppress it, me, as much.

INT: *You have choices: to open up to all the parts of yourself, including the parts of you that can offer such joy.*

CASSANDRA: I know I can feel so sexy, because music makes me feel sexy and I fantasize about music in my mind when I have sex. It sort of breaks down my walls and carries me away from the "good-girl" or "bad-girl stuff." It's just *me* and I feel happy. I love hearing my lover's voice and I tell him to talk to me. I really love that! But even if he doesn't talk to me, I can hear whatever words I need to hear if I let myself relax and focus on some of the words in the Michael Bolton songs. Before I make love I can get more relaxed by putting on my music and then carrying it in my head when we make love.

I don't think he knows there's a musical
accompaniment to our lovemaking, [laughs] but
so what? It really sends me.

INT: *So the part of you that you've been calling
outrageous is the wonderful part, the alive and
creative part, the part that you've been keeping
underground may be the very best part of all. From
what you say, it sounds like it is time for you
to rethink this and realize that it's good to have
fun—to rediscover and celebrate the best parts of
you.*

CASSANDRA: I never thought of it as a choice, or
that I already had what I needed. I really
didn't. I thought I had to find a partner who didn't
put up walls. It's so hard finding the ideal partner.
This guy is wonderful in so many ways—not
perfect—but great. I can see that my fun has
really more to do with me and that I've been more
interested in him or anticipating his reactions
and not what I like, like nature, or music.

INT: *How do you feel when you think about having
these choices for yourself?*

CASSANDRA: A lot more free to act on my inner feelings
and to have my fantasies without feeling badly.
I'm sure it will take some practice, but I'm
ready to try something different. If I think about
my music, I guess I've learned how to tune out
other people and focus on music instead. I'm
going to practice doing the same thing at
other times—just acting spontaneously and not
laboring over my decisions or what others will

think. As I get older, I tell myself, "What are you waiting for? You're middle-aged and you deserve more sexual joy in your life." I feel ready to begin to give myself permission to feel better in many ways. I think I might really be happy—or choose to be happy—much more often.

Cassandra has strengths in Clusters 2 and 3. She can lose herself in music and, during those times, let go of any critical awareness that can stop the flow. She is also able to lose herself in daydreams (Cluster 5) and can easily access vivid memories from her past (Cluster 4) while listening to music. But sexually, she is easily distracted by thoughts of being "bad" and is not able to focus on what she loves. Thus, Cluster 1 is an area she identified for enhancement. She recognized the need to learn to redefine the good-bad split, and reconnect with pleasure. She can also develop her cross-sensory enjoyment (Cluster 6) by listening to her favorite music and imagining what colors or textures the notes and melodies would be. As she deepens all of her clusters and embraces joy more readily—as a woman, and not as a little girl—she will find herself more immersed in supersexual passion.

Colleen, a forty-one-year-old physical therapist with two children, is a medium-high absorber who scored 20 on the absorption scale and has gotten in touch with many qualities in her supersexual nature. She takes responsibility for her own feelings, delights in her vivid imagination, and immerses herself in a novel with ease. She can experience supersex sometimes, but not always. She agreed to a follow-up interview because she wanted to understand what it was about herself that contributed to limiting her joy. "It feels so terrific when I'm lost in sex—I want to learn to be there more often!" At the time of this interview, Colleen was seven months pregnant and feeling wonderful about the prospect of having another child.

INT: *Tell me about an especially happy moment in your life.*

COLLEEN: It's talking and sharing with others. I really don't find happiness in huge events; for me, it's in each moment. Sometimes even in the middle of all my daily stress, I have moments when I feel "really me." I'm basically impulsive: when something feels good—all things being okay—I do it. What I love to do is to get together with friends and just laugh—to the point where I actually get lost in whatever we are doing together. Laughing with people I love is a real release for me. I take great pleasure in it.

INT: *Have you always been someone who gets lost in things easily?*

COLLEEN: Absolutely. As a child I can remember getting lost in some comic book at the grocery store and forgetting to pick up the things my mother asked me to get. Even now I get totally lost in my reading. I am highly empathic: I identify with the character so much, I sometimes get depressed at the end of a book. I choose what I will read or watch on TV because I empathize so deeply that they can really upset me. I prefer some drama or comedy with warm, close relationships.

INT: *What is it that you like best about your ability to empathize?*

COLLEEN: I just like the feel of connecting—of interacting—whether it's with people or with characters in a book, play, or movie. I'm not a person who likes brain teasers or mind-games in books—I like the feeling of that interpersonal connection. It's almost like there is an invisible thing that happens when I connect, and if I can feel that and move with it, it doesn't matter what the outcome is. I'm not outcome oriented—I just enjoy being part of something that interests me.

INT: *How does that interest—and the importance of connecting to what interests you—bridge to sexuality?*

COLLEEN: I don't think I would want to have really absorbing sex with someone who I didn't feel connected to interpersonally—that casual sex experience. Maybe I could—but I don't think I would want that for myself. The times that I have had sex without emotional connection, even with an orgasm, wasn't as much fun. I would have to find the whole process, the person and the situation, interesting.

INT: *Are you aware of how you make it interesting?*

COLLEEN: Well, I guess that's true—I do make it interesting when I make a decision about when I will or won't let go. I have even awakened from a dream and felt that I have had an orgasm

in my sleep, just from my thoughts. So I know
that I can give myself pleasure—even without
a partner. I just prefer doing it with a partner.

INT: *What does the partner have to do with it for you?*

COLLEEN: Without a partner, the physical sensations
just aren't as intense. I like having his body
to experience along with my own. I guess he
has to be there and I have to feel fairly secure
with him before I can let go.

INT: *What else keeps you from letting go sexually?*

COLLEEN: I guess I'd call them inhibitions. For
me, some of my inhibitions are body inhibitions.
I have only had one partner for several years
now—my husband. But even as a young
woman, I think I might have been more
sexually active, selectively, of course, if I'd felt
more comfortable with my body. I grew up fat,
so I had a lot of fears about people making
fun of my body. I still need some reassurance
that my body isn't ugly. I know that my husband
doesn't think my body is ugly and I trust him.
I also know that I feel safe with him, but in
my own mind—when I fantasize—I want a
body that is acceptable to my partner.

INT: *How do you feel about the changes in your body
during your pregnancy?*

COLLEEN: I enjoy the changes in my body,
surprisingly. I guess it's because it's a time when
it's expected that my body will get larger. There's

something freeing about that. I feel very feminine and sensual. My breasts and nipples are more sensitive when I'm pregnant and when I have an orgasm I can feel my uterus contract.

INT: *What senses and images do you enjoy during sex?*

COLLEEN: I enjoy the smells of my partner's body—the ordinary perspiration. I have never been one of those people who need to shower before sex. I don't like perfumes that cover the natural smells. I've always liked sexual imagery and looking at sensual pictures, too. I suppose that I have always appreciated a bodily perspective in sexuality. But when I'm not pregnant, thoughts about the acceptability of my own body sometimes distract me.

INT: *Do you think these thoughts place limits on your sexual pleasure?*

COLLEEN: Yes, I think so. I have always liked keeping the lights really low during lovemaking because I've never felt comfortable with people looking at me. As a teenager, a lot of guys admired my large breasts, and I thought, "Maybe they'll just look there and not notice my big thighs or my overweight stomach." [Laughs.] I've always been big in a society that hasn't valued large women. It's been a difficult adjustment. I enjoy watching pornographic films, but I don't like to be watched. Even though I'm comfortable with my husband, when he stares at me while I'm dressing or

undressing, it's not entirely comfortable. I
sometimes wonder what he's thinking and if
my body is pleasing to him.

INT: *So you pay attention to his thoughts and wonder*
if he's thinking or feeling something negative about
your body?

COLLEEN: Right. It can be really unsettling and
a turn-off for me.

INT: *Have you thought about how you can get beyond*
this inhibition? Are there ways you have found
to minimize your concern?

COLLEEN: Yes. It's back to where we started, really.
When I allow myself to let go to whatever interests
me—a book or a conversation with friends—
and I'm really focused there, my mind is still
and I'm just aware that I'm having fun. When
we're in the middle of making love, I'm just there
with my husband and when I'm really into the
pleasure I don't think of anything else. I get
more connected to what I'm feeling because it
feels good. Once in a while a thought about my
body may jump in, but if I stay connected to
the good feeling, it just goes back to where
it came from. But I still like keeping the bedroom
lights dim: I think that's been my way to make
sex more comfortable and safe for myself.

INT: *That's been something you've consciously*
chosen to do?

COLLEEN: Yes, but I sometimes say, I wish I could just be more comfortable in the bright light and love my body more completely. I don't think enjoying sex has to do with weight. I think that women who are heavy and are comfortable with their bodies are beautiful. I think women—fat or thin—who are uptight or uncomfortable expressing themselves are less sensual and certainly having less fun! It's really more of a mind-set. I'm getting more convinced of this as we talk.

INT: *So I hear you saying that you would like—*

COLLEEN: To feel less self-conscious. And as my biological clock continues to tick, I feel more motivated to change my thinking and preoccupation with my "bad" body image. In grade school I went through years with the kids calling me "hog" and "Sherm" and a lot of it unfortunately stuck. But there's a battle inside because a part of me feels very attractive and sensual but part of me still remembers the old labels.

INT: *So you can't change your history, but you can make a choice about how much to let it influence your present life and your future.*

COLLEEN: That's true. Just verbalizing this has been helpful to me. I see how I let these old messages take up space in my life: I do make a choice to listen to them instead of doing what I enjoy. I feel that the time has come for me to worry less about how I look and to be less self-critical. I think I need to brighten the

light, so to speak, and take another look at
Colleen—to check out the reality I feel today
instead of operating from the past. I know that
I've already made a start. After my last son
was born, I threw away all my small-size clothes
because I was tired of dieting and focusing my
life on getting down to a size ten or a twelve.
I'm more comfortable with myself as a
fourteen. Sexually, I'm the same woman whether
I am a size ten or a fourteen! When I tell myself
I'm healthy, strong, sexual, and intelligent, I
feel great. Then on other days, I'm not so
sure—and those are the days that the negative
thoughts creep into my mind. There are also some
practical issues about having sex when there
are three children who need to be put to bed,
and it takes time to settle down and not be tired.
I've been doing much too much professionally
and socially. All of the logistical problems of
living in this day and age sometimes take me
away from my pleasure, too.

INT: *Yet, in the midst of your problems, there are times
when you can lose yourself in the sexual moment
and feel ecstasy.*

COLLEEN: Yes, I can! So I know that I can do it
regardless of these externals I've been listing (as
real as they are). Actually, the way I got
pregnant this time was that I was so deeply
focused on pleasure that it was the one time I
didn't use birth control—so I'm forty-one years
old and pregnant! [Laughs.] So I know that
I can let go. I just don't do it as consistently
as I would like to. I'm not sure that I have believed

that I could actually limit the distractions that just enter my mind: they seem to have a mind of their own! It's a little different thinking that I have a choice—I feel some excitement about it. I'd like to stay on track more often and circumvent that body inhibition distraction.

INT: *The more you practice focusing on the feelings, senses, images, thoughts—whatever—that you enjoy, the more natural it will become. It's an option you can choose: you only need to notice when you go off track, and redirect your attention to what you love.*

Colleen is intermittently experiencing supersex. She responded affirmatively to questions in all the clusters and has a genuine desire to deepen her absorption in pleasure. During sex, she has only one major distraction: preoccupations with her weight, a problem she is exploring. She has a ways to go, but she is beginning to believe that a "perfect" body is not a prerequisite for sexual joy.

Questions to Ponder If You're a Medium-High Absorber

As you've seen from these interviews, developing your supersexual potential requires realization of how you both create and limit your sexual and nonsexual pleasure. If you have an Inner Critic, a negative view of pleasure, a body-image concern, or a belief that you can only find joy with the "perfect" partner, here are some questions to consider:

- Do you sometimes sense an inner debate between one inner voice (the critic) and another (the spontaneous you)?
- When these voices debate, which one wins?
- During sex, how do these voices keep you from enjoying yourself?
- Think of a time when you followed your spontaneous voice (true voice) during a moment of deep pleasure (sexual or non-sexual). What conditions, situations, feelings were important to enjoying those pleasures?
- Think about ways to maximize those pleasure-affirming thoughts, feelings, images, and senses *sexually*.

Chapter 12 will explore these questions in greater depth.

Elena: A High Absorber Who Stops Herself

Right now, some of you are no doubt thinking, "I'm scoring high on the absorption scale, so why aren't I experiencing supersex?" When a high absorber still is not enjoying supersex, it's because for some reason, she's not ready to let go. Often it's because she doesn't feel completely safe with her partner.

This was certainly true in the following case. Elena is thirty-four, works in the advertising business, and recently went through a break-up with the woman she had considered her life partner. She scored high on the absorption scale, with a score of 26. She reported high levels of absorption when reading books she loved, cooking, going to the theater, and being intensely involved in an advertising project. During orgasms with her former partner, she "felt intense sensations of color, like buttercup yellow or intense violet, and texture, like the stones of an ancient, crumbling wall ... very fleeting, momentary vision-feelings." She had heard a woman describe a supersexual experience, was interested, and came for a follow-up interview on the subject.

ELENA: I had these vivid moments, and often cried
after making love. Not from sadness, but from
something else. Sort of like spring rain. But
I never had an out-of-body experience, or
soared to the stars, or had the ability for sustained
lovemaking. I've never been multi-orgasmic, either.

INT: *What was happening for you during the vivid*
moments? Did you feel yourself able to let go?
Release into the feeling?

ELENA: I'm not sure how I would have done that.

INT: *What was the most important, most special*
thing about lovemaking for you?

ELENA: It was ... an intense emotional connection
that I felt, sometimes, with my partner. The
emotional and the physical, together. As time
went on, I continued to go for that emotional
connection, but she was approaching sex very
much as a physical activity, a workout, like going
for a run or something.

INT: *So she didn't always stay emotionally connected*
with you?

ELENA: Right. During orgasm, when I would have
these moments, I felt really alone,

disconnected from her. And then I would
come back, try to "find" her. Try to bring her
into my experience. Just, have her be with me.
But she was somewhere else most of the time.
In the beginning, she was more with me. But
looking back on it, now I can see that she was
detached, sexually, and I kept seeking her.

INT: *It sounds to me like you pulled back, stopped yourself
from moving into what we call supersexual
experience. You know, a lot of people don't put
as much value on that continued emotional
connectedness with a partner. So it's easier for them
to release, physically, during a potentially supersexual
moment. For you, it would have been a denial
of who you are and what you value to
"transcend" supersexually without her. It's a conscious
protective choice you made. She may be a low
absorber, very reliant and comfortable with her
boundaries, keeping you out, emotionally. That
was her choice. In a way you were at cross-purposes—
she was closing off sexually and emotionally while
you wanted to open up.*

ELENA: So we had a high absorber, me, trying
to have supersex with a somewhat low absorber,
and it wasn't working. We weren't in sync.

INT: *Exactly. I think that the fact that you were able
to let go and see colors and textures with the
person is evidence of your supersexual potential and
passion.*

This high absorber is, most likely, on the verge of
supersexual experience. She scored high in many of the

absorption clusters. Emotional connection is so important to her that until she finds a partner who can sustain that kind of connectedness and considers her own readiness to let go, it's doubtful that she will allow herself to supersexually transcend.

In the next chapter, you will discover more about the supersexual mind-set, and about how to enhance your capacity—and readiness—for supersexual pleasure.

∽ CHAPTER 12 ∽

The Supersexual Mind-Set

*"Would you tell me, please, which way I ought
to go from here?"
"That depends a good deal on where you want
to get to," said the cat.
"I don't much care where," said Alice.
"Then it doesn't matter which way you go,"
said the cat.*

—Lewis Carroll,
Alice in Wonderland

By now you have become more aware of your own absorption clusters and your potential to immerse yourself in pleasure. This chapter takes you a step further in understanding the ingredients that are central to *all* of the absorption clusters—the supersexual mind-set.

The way we think and feel about ourselves, our partner, and our sexuality (in the broadest sense) creates our experience and definition of "erotic" pleasure. There is no absolute agreement about what constitutes an erotic experience. It varies. Whether a particular moment is felt to be a turn-on or a turn-off has less to do with the moment itself, and more to do with your state of mind—your mind-set. Think about the times when hand-holding or looking at your lover's body was enough to make you melt, and another time when sexual intercourse left you cold. What made the difference? Which situation was more sensual or sexual for you? You may not have realized it, but you control how you experience pleasure by your choices (conscious and unconscious). You have the ability to enhance or deepen your pleasure if you choose to.

Women learn to access pleasure differently, across all of their clusters. We've stressed the importance of psychological absorption because what you experience depends on what you notice and how deeply you notice it. By changing your focus of attention, you also change your experience. Are we suggesting that there is no absolutely perfect sexual technique or way to ring his/her bells every time? Exactly. No one can give you or your partner sexual ecstasy; it is there for the taking if you are open to it. Freeing yourself of distractions, and redirecting your attention to what you find pleasing is central to pleasure of all kinds. Other facets of the supersexual mind-set include:

- Learning to quiet the mind
- Staying connected to what you love—letting the moment lead you
- Trusting your partner and yourself
- Finding your own "true" voice among the "shoulds"
- Suspending certainty and cultivating a beginner's mind
- Enhancing your enjoyment of senses, images, and fantasies

Taken together, these facets illustrate how supersexual women think about sexuality and access a different kind of sexual reality. Although each facet is presented separately, it cannot be understood in isolation from the rest. Just as the pattern of an intricate tapestry depends upon the relationship of each thread, the supersexual mind-set depends on a pattern of thinking that deepens all of the clusters of the absorption spectrum. Once you have explored these facets, you will be ready to consider building your ecstasy connection in Chapter 13.

Learning to Quiet the Mind

We know from our research that women who permit themselves to quiet their minds and to experience a relaxed focus on internal self-generated images or fantasies report more intense sexual arousal. Being able to redirect the conscious mind as you would in a meditative or hypnotic trance is one key to discovering sexual ecstasy. Although meditation is a well-known pathway to the inner self, it is not a shortcut to supersex. The inner focus achieved during meditation and the relaxed concentration these women report during supersex are similar in many ways, but they are not interchangeable. It is true that a certain level of calmness and relaxed focus accompanies supersexual passion and that many supersexual women *do* practice some form of meditation—if not during sex, certainly at other times in their lives. "I do self-hypnosis and a lot of times when I feel the stress of the day is too much for me, I'll sit in a recliner chair and just blank out," Adelle says. "I don't care what's on TV or if the phone rings, I don't even notice ... it's like I just take a mini-vacation. And when I come back, I feel better."

Several women also spoke of using some form of meditation to get in the mood before making love. Felicia says, "Let me put it this way. I have learned how to go 'fuzzy' ... it's a kind of right-hemisphere unfocused visualizing. And I can pretty much do that at will. How? I relax my body, breathe everything I need into my body and then exhale my stress, and then let my eyes gently close. You kind of half-lid your eyes and allow the experience of relaxation to come to you. They talk about this in Buddhism. I think that it puts me in a place to have the experience, if it's to be had."

Thich Nhat Hanh, a Vietnamese Buddhist poet and teacher, offers an approach to emptying our minds to allow a present-centered awareness to enter our consciousness. He instructs us to open to life by reciting the following poem while breathing and smiling:

> Breathing in, I calm body and mind.
> Breathing out, I smile
> Dwelling in the present moment
> I know this is the only moment

There are a number of excellent resources available to help you quiet your mind. You may read Herbert Benson's *Relaxation Response* or find comfort in reciting a favorite prayer. Or you might try the guided imagery we have included in the appendix as a way to relax your mind. It doesn't really matter which method you choose. What matters is that you select one that feels right for you and that you practice it until you can relax easily and comfortably. Not all supersexual women meditate, per se. Some of them have "naturally" learned a sort of mindful silence and relaxed concentration or receptivity that allows supersex to emerge. Once you have quieted your mind, you will be ready to open to what you love.

Staying Connected to What You Love— Letting the Moment Lead You

We all know that we make deliberate choices about how to spend our weekend, or whether to buy that new car. But we are often unaware of the less-than-conscious choices we make moment by moment that affect the quality of our sexual connections. By operating on "automatic pilot" we miss many opportunities for sexual pleasure and lovemaking can become routine. Staying connected to what you love and letting the moment lead you sounds so simple, until you think about how often we separate ourselves from our feelings.

Consider how many times you may have kissed your partner hello or good-bye and not really "been there." You may have been going through the motions in some perfunctory manner—without noticing any feelings or sensations. It is as if you have removed part of your awareness. Your lips are there, but the rest of you (emotions, spirit) has gone somewhere else. But where have you gone? Perhaps, as you kiss good-bye, your mind is considering the next task on your daily agenda: will the children be ready in time to catch the school bus? Whatever occupies your mind, it carries you away from your pleasure.

You might be saying, "But there are realities in life—there is so much to do and so little time!" Yes, but does it take more time to notice that kiss in a pleasurable way, or is it just deciding to stay connected? This absent-minded, automatic way of kissing good-bye or repeating, "I love you too," is often the way many couples make love. Their bodies may be there, but the rest of them has gone somewhere else. How can sexuality be pleasurable if *you* aren't there? In supersex, the women we studied stay very connected to their passion and allow it to lead them somewhere pleasurable and ecstatic.

Think once again of your lovemaking. Do you find your mind wandering to worries about the bills, or whether he's going to lose his erection or come too fast? Or whether your partner will get tired during oral sex before you're ready to come? Are you paying attention to what *you* like, or just what your partner likes? Do you take time to notice what feels good to you? If you'd like to practice letting the moment lead you, next time you make love, pay special attention to what you love and say to yourself internally, "I really *like* the way the pressure of his body *feels* right now, or the smell of his skin, or the sound of his breathing, or

the tingling I feel when I hear those passionate words."
Make the feelings more explicit for yourself. Notice what
memories, images, or feelings enter your mind and trust in
yourself to let the pleasurable experiences guide you.

But what about the mind chatter—how can you minimize the worries and distractions that seem to intrude at
the most inopportune times? When confronted with inevi-
table anxieties or concerns—thoughts that interrupt the
pleasure focus—supersexual women have learned to notice the distraction, comment on it briefly, and then refocus their attention to what they enjoy. So, if you are in the
midst of a passionate moment and you find an unwelcome
thought entering your consciousness, just acknowledge it
to yourself, "O.K. I've just gotten distracted," and then redirect your focus to what you like—to the touch, the
smells, the tastes, the look, or to your pleasurable images
or fantasies. Don't fight the distractions or try to block
them out—you know how hard it is to *not* think of a pink
elephant. Just acknowledge the break in your focus and let
it go.

At work or play, take time to notice what you like. The
comfortable fit of a favorite tool in your hand, the sight of
a leaf moving in the breeze, the smoothness of your partner's skin—such simple pleasures keep you in touch with
your passion. By staying connected to what you love, you
are allowing your *pleasure* to become the guiding force
that will direct you across all absorption clusters to the experience of supersex.

Trusting Your Partner and Yourself

The ability to open to supersex depends on a trusting relationship with your partner and a feeling of safety.
Supersexual women open to passion only when they feel

safe and comfortable letting go. When you feel uncomfortable, whatever the reason, it is as if there is a watchful, protective eye that holds you back and keeps you in check. By holding back, you choose not to cross that imaginary boundary that separates you from supersex. You may have felt a similar boundary in other aspects of your sexual response. Perhaps there are times when you feel close to having an orgasm but have difficulty letting yourself cross over into it. Some women know this boundary very well. The harder you try, the more elusive your orgasm becomes. You learn to orgasm by following that internal wave of joy and merging with it. The boundary between satisfactory sex and supersex is similar to the one you approach before orgasm, and the process is the same. It involves choosing to follow your pleasure and to deepen it—beyond orgasm.

If this experience is so wonderful, why doesn't everyone simply open up their boundaries and merge with joy? Because the choices to hold back are often intelligent, protective decisions—especially in relationships where there has been a breach of trust. Some women feel uncomfortable opening to themselves because of low self-esteem, discomfort with their body image, or a range of other feelings that affect their sexual comfort. Other women only feel constrained with certain partners and not others. These women discover that they can easily let go while masturbating or with a safe lover.

Women have many reasons for holding back. Bethaney, a thirty-two-year-old homemaker, is married to Art, a forty-eight-year-old postal clerk whom she describes as "basically a good man, but with a sarcastic sense of humor." She was born in Poland in a strict, traditional home and was taught that her feelings came second to her husband's. As the oldest daughter of nine siblings, she was "always there for everyone else," she says, "but I suppose

I never thought about what I wanted or needed." Recently, she began to feel that something was wrong with her marriage and her sexual relationship. She came to therapy because she discovered that she could be orgasmic during masturbation, but not with her husband. She wanted to be happier with him. "In my home in Poland I can remember my mother telling me to overlook things and not argue—Art and I don't argue—but I feel hurt by some of his comments. He makes them seem like jokes, but they're not funny to me."

Bethaney and Art don't struggle openly. That's one of their problems. She feels hurt by his hostility but has been afraid to tell him—afraid things would get worse if she did. During sex she was holding herself back in a protective way. "One time," she said sadly, "I think I was close to having an orgasm and he laughed at me, saying I looked foolish—like a panting dog. He also makes comments about my hygiene and I'm not sure if he's being serious. I just don't feel comfortable being myself with Art—it's sad."

Both Bethaney and Art were involved in creating an unsafe environment for sexual expression. They had a number of issues to discuss and resolve. Art's hostility and sarcasm bordered on emotional abuse. Bethaney had to find the courage to go against her earlier messages to overlook problems and to now trust her feelings. When she became more honest with Art, he began to listen. As they each learned to more openly disagree and express their feelings to each other in therapy, his hostility and her compliance diminished. He learned to recognize and take responsibility for his hurtful "playfulness" and deal more directly with his anger. She began to protect herself by not accepting Art's hurtful comments, to define her sexuality in ways that were comfortable to her, and to feel freer to experience more joy in her sexual relationship. Over time, with practice in being self-protective and self-assertive,

Bethaney's trust in their relationship gradually improved. Not long after, she was able to achieve orgasm with Art when she desired it.

When you think about your own partner, pay attention to when you can comfortably let go to pleasure. What does it depend upon? Consider what it would take for you to feel safe now. Once you have decided, the next step is to move in the direction of creating more safety for yourself.

Finding Your Own "True" Voice Among the "Shoulds"

Another aspect of enhancing your absorption clusters is learning to recognize your own "true" voice among a myriad of internalized "shoulds." Trying to please the many voices that often echo in our minds is a sure-fire way to limit our sexual joy. These voices may take many forms—those of mentors, parents, friends, media messages, among others. If they clash—and they usually do—you may feel pushed or pulled in a variety of directions.

Alice Miller, an analyst who has written extensively on children's adaptations to parental needs, writes:

> Accommodation to parental needs often (but not always) leads to the "as if personality." (Winnicott has described it as the "false self.") This person develops in such a way that he reveals only what is expected of him and fuses so completely with what he reveals ... that one could scarcely have guessed how much more there is to him. He cannot develop and differentiate his "True self" because he is unable to live it.
> —Alice Miller, *The Drama of the Gifted Child*

When it comes to sex, there are many messages to sort through from a lifetime of ideas, values, attitudes, myths, and often misconceptions, cultural and religious teachings, etc., about what should be "right," "normal," or "healthy" for you. If your earliest experience with intimacy as a young child was being sexually fondled by your next-door neighbor, it will set the stage for you to consider sexuality as hurtful and confusing. Each of our experiences shapes our beliefs about our own sexuality and intrinsic goodness.

Fortunately, life affords us opportunities to modify our views—to check in with ourselves often to see if we still ascribe to the same ideas, feelings, or attitudes we once believed. Supersexual women recognize that sexual growth, along with all other human development, is a lifelong process. Attempting to struggle with these internalized voices of authority and reconcile them with your own true voice is a critical aspect of maturation and sexual self-discovery. As you continue to open yourself to a richer sexual experience, it would be useful for you to identify your own sexual "shoulds" or prohibitions. Think about whose voice comes to you and whether those messages still feel "true" to you.

Your attitudes and beliefs about sexuality direct your choices while you are making love. They may come in the form of distracting voices urging you to perform according to some unrealistic or perfectionistic standard. Or they may stem from a need for approval, fear of disappointing your partner, or countless other "shoulds" that crowd our bedrooms and our minds. When you make love, who else have you inadvertently invited in with you? Is your mother or father watching? Perhaps they have told you that they want grandchildren and you feel pressured to oblige them. How about your teachers or the pastor of the church; do their messages conflict with anything you would like to experience? How do you remedy that situation? It's impossible to pay attention to your own pleasure and to the other voices simultaneously. If there is a struggle, which voice wins?

Often, to minimize anxiety, we may deny that there is a struggle. We just limit any new information that challenges our beliefs. This practice follows the old "ignorance is bliss" adage. You could simply say, "this is the way *I* feel," and ignore anything that might challenge your beliefs. You can readily see how this solution leads to a dead end. What you believe directs your choices, and by closing your mind to new thinking, you close the door to supersex.

Think of your mind as a screen or a filtering device. The filter is made up of the internalized "shoulds" you carry about sexuality and pleasure. All new experience must pass through these internalized voices, and they are either allowed in or screened out of consciousness. If the "shoulds" are overly restrictive, the holes in the screen are small and only a limited amount of new experience is allowed through. For example, if you believe it is a wife's duty to please her husband and that sex is *not* to be enjoyed, you may have sexual intercourse out of obligation and feel guilty if there is any accompanying pleasure. Or if you have been taught that genitals are "dirty," then you may avoid oral sex. Consider your own history and the choices you have made about your sexuality. Have you limited your options in significant ways by restricting what you feel, think, imagine, or participate in? Have you learned to listen to other voices to the exclusion of your own? If so, you may have unwittingly obstructed the wisdom that is inside. Perhaps it is time to challenge your views by taking a fresh look—to open that cognitive screen. By doing so, you may discover everything that was around you all the time but that you simply hadn't seen yet. The good news is that you have the choice to modify and open your alternatives at any time. When you do choose to move in the direction of less restrictive thoughts, feelings, and behaviors—regardless of how small a move it is—you begin to actively change your experience in a positive way.

Suspending Certainty and Cultivating a Beginner's Mind

Before you are ready to enjoy supersex, you must be interested in suspending your certainty long enough to look at yourself and your partner in fresh, original ways, as if you were seeing each other for the first time. Too often, we assume that we already know what our partner's skin feels like, where and how we like to be touched, what time is best for making love, and so on. By assuming what each lovemaking session will be like, avenues for newness are closed off.

Often, when asked to describe what she feels when she touches her partner's skin, a sex therapy client will reply, "His chest felt the way it *always* does," as if the experience never changes for her. But we all know that the way we experience any pleasure, from food to music, *does* change as our sensitivities shift. Whether or not we're in the mood has a lot to do with how good a touch may feel. It's similar to going to the supermarket when you're hungry and everything looks tempting! We are, in reality, always changing, and our interests, preferences, and sensory experiences vary. When it's 100 degrees and humid outside, your lovemaking will feel very different than when you're close together beneath a down comforter in mid-winter. At times you may want sex to be hard and quick, at other times lingering and gentle. Sometimes your lover's skin may smell and taste salty. Another time, it may smell freshly clean and slightly scented with soap. When you're open to all of these nuances, you begin to realize you *don't* really know what to expect from one sexual moment to the next—that each moment you're making love offers an infinite range of fresh, exciting possibilities.

But there is a kind of comfort in believing that we "know" with certainty what will work each time, and that we have somehow mastered the techniques perfectly. What often happens is that routine, predictable sex leads to boredom. It's also not true that certain techniques work every time, or can be repeated in some rote manner. Have you ever tried to repeat an especially intense romantic moment by doing everything the same way you did before? You may light the candles, pour the drinks, put on the music, return to the same vacation spot, touch the same erogenous zones, but somehow, this time the magic doesn't happen. Why not? Could it be that you missed it? The pleasure may have been there but in a different form. *By expecting the magic of the previous time, we overlook the passion of this time.* Once we open our awareness and focus on the present moment, we discover sexual pleasure is always there for us, waiting to be enjoyed.

How routine is your lovemaking? Do you think that you know what each sexual encounter will probably be like? Can you predict where you'll have sex, what time of day or night, or what day of the week? Do you know who will initiate and how it will end? If you can answer yes to any of these questions, then you have cultivated a certainty about your sexual relationship which can be limiting your experiences. Now you might say, "But I *do* know how it's going to be—it's been that way for years!" Yes, and it's a self-fulfilling prophecy; you usually get what you expect and find what you're looking for. You also only experience what you notice. As soon as you begin to suspend your certainty and cultivate a beginner's mind, anything becomes possible and sex is always new and exciting.

Supersexual women have learned to approach each moment with an openness to experience and a state of conscious awareness that pushes against boundaries we have learned to think of as conventional. By trusting their intuition and following their emotions, they have learned to cultivate a spiritual richness and sensitivity to connections which sometimes defy description. Many of them have felt "touched" at the very center of their being by learning to trust the passion from within.

Prudence, a vibrant sixty-year-old divorced woman in the publishing business, describes supersex with her lover of the past eighteen years as "communication from soul to soul. It's so exciting that our loving stays so fresh after all these years. I don't expect anything in particular; I guess I just go with whatever happens each time. Sometimes I begin to have these lovely fantasies that I follow. All I can say is that I have felt a spiritual connection that moves me beyond words!" Prudence is a high absorber and has accessed all of the clusters of the absorption spectrum. "What's most amazing," she says with delight, "is that it keeps getting better."

Walt Whitman referred to this altered state of conscious awareness in his poem "Miracles" when he wrote of seeing everything in life—"every cubic inch" and "every hour of the light and dark"—as a miracle. "After all," Whitman once told a friend, "the great lesson is that no special natural sight—not the Alps, Niagara Falls, or Yosemite, or anything else—is more grand or beautiful than the ordinary sunrise and sunset, earth and sky, the common trees and grass." Like the poet, supersexual women know that the grandest experiences in life are no lovelier, finer, nor better than the commonplace and what we really need to enjoy life is to become sensitive to the neverending sources of wonder all around and within us.

Replacing certainty with erotic curiosity allows you to discover newness in the same partner time after time by cultivating a "beginner's mind." In other words, approach every sexual interlude as if it were the first. This may sound odd, but it merely requires a bit of practice. Don't jump ahead of yourself—just keep pace with what you notice through your senses. Whatever erotic thoughts and images emerge, follow them. Respond spontaneously and naturally, without much "analytical" thought. Take a familiar part of your partner's body and explore it as if you have never seen it before. Touch a variety of skin surfaces, be creative, and notice what you discover. Is touching with your fingertips different from touching with your hand, or with your lips? Remember that your sensations will change, and that each moment provides a new opportunity for further discovery. When you look at your partner, what do you see? Remember the passion of that first kiss? Recreate the feeling in your mind. Now kiss again—not to compare, just to enjoy.

As supersexual women have continually pointed out, direct experience does not easily translate into words or set rules. Noting that the English language is particularly bereft of color words, Diane Ackerman, author of *The Language of the Senses,* says that if we want our language to reflect what [high absorbers] can truly see: "We need to boost our range of greens to describe the almost squash-yellow of late winter grass, the achingly fluorescent green of the leaves of high summer and all the whims of chlorophyll in between. We need words for the many colors of clouds, surging from pearly pink during a calm sunset over the ocean to the electric gray-green of tornadoes. An apple remains red in our minds whenever we see it, but think how different its red looks under a fluorescent light, on the shady branch of a tree, on a patio at night, or in a knapsack."

Just as a fish cannot appreciate the feeling of wetness because it has never felt dry, we who are lost in the certainty of our mind-set have difficulty cultivating a fresh sexual perspective. Cultivating a beginner's mind challenges you to transcend the boundaries you have become accustomed to—those limiting messages, standards, ideals, and beliefs about what one needs to be or have to enjoy passionate sexuality. By re-examining the terrain, you will discover a range of possibilities difficult to categorize, but delightful to experience. It will permit you to explore your passion across all of the absorption clusters—to enhance your arousal, imagery, memories, emotions, sensory pleasures, and spiritual connection. When experienced this way, lovemaking does not grow dull with the same partner year after year, because it's always as if you're making love for the first time.

Enhancing Your Enjoyment of
Senses, Images, and Fantasies

The last facet of the supersexual mind-set is learning to discover and expand your sensory enjoyment. Perhaps more than any other psychological process, your sensory imagery and sensory appreciations are uniquely your own. They have evolved over a lifetime through a variety of experiences. Some say we are born with a certain capacity for imagery, while others say it is learned. The most generally endorsed view, which we share, is that the capacity for imagery is modified by learning and that this learning is neverending. Your images and sensory awareness are your personal connections to all of the possibilities that lie within you. Over the decades, images, daydreams, fantasies, and sensory experiences have been defined in a variety of ways. We are using the term *image* to define any thought that has a sensory quality and occurs in the absence of the actual sensation. Through your images, you can recall the sensual feeling of running your hand through your lover's hair. The more vividly you are able to imagine this, the more pleasurable the feeling can become. Some people say that they cannot imagine or fantasize. If you can visualize a red square and then turn it into a blue square or a yellow square, you have just experienced visual imagery. If you can recall the sound of the wheels of a train, the smell of bacon, the aroma of your lover's cologne, you are using auditory and olfactory imagery. If you were asked how many doors or windows there are in your home, you rely on your imagery to answer that question.

The words *imagery* and *fantasy* are often used interchangeably. An image or fantasy can include a brief daydream or flickering image which appears as you are driving your car along some familiar road, or a full-length erotic movie which you replay in your mind. During sleep, your imagery takes the form of dreams, though you may not recall them. As Shakespeare said, "We are such stuff as dreams are made of." What we imagine and how we imagine affects our conscious reality.

Researchers have not always agreed that sexual fantasy heightens arousal. In the early literature on sexuality, many writers thought that any form of sexual fantasy was an indication of dysfunction or repressed desires. Wilhelm Reich (1942) referred to sexual fantasies during intercourse as "escape mechanisms" which were diversionary distractions. These views are not supported in most scientific circles, and the more current research, including my own (Scantling, 1990), has found that women who enjoy their sexual imagery report more intense pleasure during masturbation and partner sex.

Imagery opens up tremendous possibilities in many areas. Research in sports psychology has suggested that the systematic practice of visualizing the perfect golf or tennis swing vastly improves an athlete's performance. Individual athletes have reported that they have realized significant improvement in their athletic performance by using imagery rehearsal.

When you run or swim, cook a meal, listen to a symphony, or work on your favorite project, do you experience moments when you may become so immersed and absorbed in the activity that all else may temporarily cease to exist? If so, you are well on the road to supersex. You may notice while watching an especially compelling movie that you enter the storyline and may even become a character, replete with emotion. If you have been moved to tears or laughter by a movie, no doubt you have experienced absorption. While reading a novel, you may *become* a character in the book and mentally transport yourself into the setting. Absorption is the key which allows you to enjoy the sensory richness and imagery all around and within you. By absorbing yourself in your images with the vividness and clarity you are capable of, you will awaken your potential to enjoy a surprising palette of intensity and passion which may have gone unnoticed.

By enjoying their daydreams, some women are able to recapture sexual passion that lets supersex unfold. During sex, Emma takes herself back to a special time she spent at the ocean: "When I'm making love, I usually go to the same place in my mind. It's a special spot near the ocean that I visited nearly ten years ago on vacation. I remember that the sand felt smooth—like talcum powder between my toes—and the water was this incredibly deep clear blue-green. I can get myself to relax by just thinking about it now. Smelling the clean cool air and lying on the warm sand, I can hear the waves hitting the rocks along the shore and find myself relaxing with each wave. When I'm making love, sometimes right before orgasm, my vision of the beach just goes away and is suddenly replaced by a flash of blues and purples."

It's apparent from reading this passage that Emma has the capacity to access imagery across many senses—not just visually, but through her tactile, auditory, and olfactory senses. As you expand your imagery repertoire across many senses, you learn to deepen the cluster of cross-sensory experience.

So how can you learn to enhance your own sensory repertoire? First, you need to identify your current sensory style so that you can discover ways to expand your sensory options.

To identify and explore the sensory and imagery aspects of absorption, take a moment to just relax and clear your mind—a moment for yourself. Select fifteen or twenty minutes when you have nothing pressing for your attention and no chance of interruption. Shut the ringer off on your telephone. Now, permit yourself to recall an especially pleasurable moment—any moment that captured your attention completely. Select a moment which engaged your sense of sight, smell, hearing, touch, or taste. Perhaps it was when you were swimming, or sailing, or skiing, or during a walk in the woods, or when you were cooking, or at work involved in a special project. Perhaps you will think of a moment during vacation or with your lover. Whatever the moment, allow yourself to recall this scene with as much clarity and detail as possible. Notice all aspects of the moment and, as if you were photographing the event, take time to use your zoom lens to focus in on all of the subtleties or nuances you can recall. Take as much time as you need to notice all of the sights, sounds, smells, touches, tastes, or feelings which are most vivid as you reflect on this especially pleasurable time.

Once you have completed this experience, write (or dictate) as complete a description as you can. Pay attention to the adjectives, adverbs, or verbs you use to convey the feelings you have just experienced. If any images or metaphors spontaneously come to mind, record them also. By looking at the words you used to describe the experience, you will be able to get some clues to your sensory absorption.

For example, let's assume that you imagined skiing down a mountain with softly packed snow on a bright clear winter's day. You could feel the cool air on your face and felt exhilarated as you sped down the slope. Using just this much, we can identify that the "softly packed snow" is a kinesthetic sense. The "bright clear winter's day" is visual. "Feeling" the cool air is tactile, and so on. What is not present in this description is an auditory sensation. You are multi-sensorial, but may choose to develop your auditory senses to further expand your pleasure. You might do this by closing your eyes while watching TV to heighten your reliance on auditory information.

To help yourself extract your sensory preferences, ask yourself the following questions:

- Are you a visual person? When you think of an idea, do you usually see pictures in your mind's eye? When you look forward to a sexual moment, do you visualize yourself with your partner? Can you visualize your partner's body clearly in its absence? How important is "seeing" your lover during sex? Do you prefer to make love with the lights on? When asking for directions, do you prefer that someone draw you a map, or would you rather get a list of directions? How important is eye contact to you? In school, did you remember instructions better if they were written on the board? How clearly can you picture an image such as the sun setting below the horizon?

- How kinesthetic or tactile (sensitive to movement and touch) are you? When you wear certain clothes, are you aware of the fabric's texture next to your skin? In stores, do you find yourself "handling" the merchandise to get a feeling for it? Are you especially sensitive to bodily sensations and do you have a low pain threshold? Is the movement or rhythm of sexuality something you can easily recall? Are you sensitive to overly starched sheets or different pillows at motels—do they interfere with your comfort or sleep? Do you experience motion sickness while traveling? How clearly can you sense your lover's touch or body against yours?

- How sensitive are you to sounds? When you hear music, are you able to discern the individual instruments, or do you tend to tune music or noises out? Do you find sounds of the ocean or the rain engaging, or are you hardly aware of them? When you make love, how important is it for you to hear words or sounds from your partner? If you wish, can you recall a favorite melody in your mind right now?

- What about your olfactory sense—your sensitivity to smells? Can certain aromas or scents, such as the smell of your partner's skin, remind you of loving times? Can just the scent bring you back to that moment? Would you be able to recognize your lover through scent alone? Are there fragrances which evoke sensual images for you?

- Finally, how sensitive are you to tastes? Do you heavily season your food, or do you prefer their natural subtle flavors? Does morning breath absolutely preclude lovemaking for you? Do you pay attention to

the taste of your partner during sex? Can certain
tastes call forth erotic or pleasurable times?

The wider your sensory repertoire, the more open you
will be to a broad range of cues—erotic and non-erotic. If
you are interested in expanding your sensory abilities, you
can practice supplementing your dominant modes. Set
aside a few minutes to focus on the less dominant senses
and soon they will be part of your attentional focus. For example, if you tend to be an auditory person, you may find
you can absorb yourself in the sounds of your lover's
breathing, your partner's voice, or music playing in the
background. You might recall in Chapter 11 that Cassandra was able to set aside her worries that her lover would
find her "outrageous" by immersing herself in music. Another supersexual woman with a highly developed auditory sense often hears soft music which lulls her into a
relaxed focus of awareness during sex.

You can adapt this strategy to any sense you enjoy. If
you're more visual than auditory, for example, you can let
go and lose yourself most easily by focusing on what you
see or imagine seeing in your mind while making love.
You might heighten your arousal by making love in front
of a mirror.

If you're a tactile person, not very visual, and usually
touch in the dark, you might develop your visual sensitivity. Begin by touching in the dark while focusing on all the
sensations, textures, temperature changes of the skin, or
contours—pay attention to whatever you find interesting.
Impress the sensations into your mind. When you are interested in expanding your sensory focus, light a candle or
dim a light and pay attention to how your experience
changes. What do you notice now? How does your experience of touching your partner's skin change with the addition of the visual sense? Practice experimenting with all of

your senses in this way. Look for the differences, because no two experiences are ever exactly the same.

That's not to suggest that we have only one sensory avenue that is dominant. Many women are able to easily access many senses. If you are interested, you can learn to notice the senses you may have been ignoring. If you tend to ignore tastes, you can focus on the way a piece of toast sweetens in your mouth as it becomes moist, or the crispness of a fresh apple, or the taste of a kiss. If you have no difficulty noticing the smell of pine needles, you can focus on the texture of the tree bark to broaden your sensory repertoire. When you are with your partner, notice the senses that you enjoy and experiment with others. Remember that your sensory preferences are your own unique composite and will vary from time to time.

A supersexual mind-set will enhance your absorption across all clusters. You are now ready to build your ecstasy connection to supersex.

CHAPTER 13

Building Your Ecstasy Connection

*There is something within every human being
that is ... the very source of all our potential; it
is the seed from which our lives grow. It is the
origin of every experience we have ever had of
love, truth, or beauty ... and it can be experienced directly.... The biggest surprise in my
search for the inner self was finding that it
could be experienced by any human being
whenever the desire was sufficiently sincere.*

—Tim Gallwey
The Inner Game of Tennis

Now that you've identified your absorption style and considered your supersexual mind-set, how do you build your
ecstasy connection? You have already begun. Each step on
this journey has brought you closer to enjoying supersex.

Although the women you have met have experienced
supersex, they would not consider themselves "masters" at
being supersexual. They know supersexual experiences continue to unfold and cannot be predictably captured. From
them we have learned to embrace supersexual passion by
opening to it, not by attempting to master or control it.

As we each walk through an art museum or wooded
park we will notice whatever interests us. If we're searching for a particular artist or species of plant, much will be
overlooked. The same is true sexually. If we are searching
for the "ultimate orgasm," we may overlook unexpected
opportunities for pleasure.

Steps to Supersexual Joy

What you have learned about how you relate to all pleasure is your connection to ecstasy. It involves building on what you already enjoy, opening to other ways of thinking, feeling, sensing, and imagining (your supersexual mindset), deepening your absorption clusters, and transferring that joy to your sexual moments.

- **Think of what you love and what you had to do with it.** Reflect upon any experience that brings you intense pleasure. We all have such peak moments. Consider what you love about these times. Ask yourself, "How did I choose to open myself to that experience?" Take some responsibility for your joy: what did you have to do with it? When things go badly for us we may ask, "What did I do wrong?" When things go well, ask yourself, "What did I do to help create my own joy?"

- **Describe that moment as clearly as possible.** Where do you put your attention? What words or images come to mind? When you're feeling intense pleasure, what do you notice? How do you deepen your enjoyment throughout the experience? If you get distracted or interrupted, how do you get back on track?

- **Consider the senses you tune in to while you're involved in what you love.** During a peak moment of pleasure, what do you see, hear, feel, taste, or smell? We have emphasized the importance of senses and images because they are critical to deepening your absorption and intensifying your sexual pleasure.

- **Discover your pleasure pattern.** If you love the feeling of wind and the movement of a sailboat you may be someone who loves motion. If you are most immersed in the feeling of wet clay as you mold shapes on a potter's wheel, you may be very tactile. Transfer whatever you have discovered about your enjoyment of pleasure to your sexual relationship.

As we've pointed out, all peak moments share many qualities in common. So, if you've experienced a joyously flowing moment at any time in your life, you can examine the patterns of that delightful experience and use them to make your sex life more special.

The following clinical example illustrates the process of building an ecstasy connection. Mark, age thirty-one, reported having problems attaining and maintaining his erection. He had waited for that "special someone," who came along when he was twenty-nine years old, before having sex. By that time, he said, he felt as if he'd gone "past the fun" because sex had become a serious worry for him. His attitude wasn't, "Wow! At last I'm going to get to see what sex is all about," but "Gee, I hope I can do it right." And, naturally, his intense anxiety practically guaranteed that he'd have problems. Fortunately, Mark did have one passionate area in his life where he didn't worry about "doing it right": bodysurfing. During two therapy sessions, he began drawing many parallels between the ecstasy he felt while bodysurfing and the ecstasy he could learn to feel while making love. Asked how he knew he was surfing the right way—was it where he positioned his body? how he held his head?—he replied, "Of course not, I do whatever works for me. It's not at all mechanical. I just learn the rhythm of the waves and then I know when to jump onto one. If you jump too early or late, it can go by you, so you learn to flow with the energy as it grabs you. I guess that's what I'm doing wrong sexually: I'm so caught up in the 'mechanics' of sex and whether I'll have an erection or not that I miss a lot of the natural waves." He began to trace his pleasure pattern by examining what he had to learn to become a good surfer. Here, in an edited version, are the parallels he drew between one passionate experience he already knew how to enjoy (bodysurfing) and the way he could use that knowledge to connect to ecstasy. Bear in mind that Mark is not a poet (he's a tax auditor). His language reflects his deep absorption in what he loves.

I love to bodysurf because I feel at one with the surf, in the moment and totally lost. Just the anticipation of seeing the ocean and the longing I feel for the water is like waiting for a lover. When I get to the beach, I can't wait to get a glimpse of the waves and if the waves are small, I used to feel disappointed sometimes, like my lover wasn't there to greet me. When I get to the beach, I just let go to the elements. Sometimes I become so immersed in the experience that I'll ride a wave right into people because I didn't even know they were there. I keep surfing until my eyes are caked with salt. I've always thought that *heaven must be like riding that endless wave.* My timing comes from inside me. I feel so connected and at one with the ocean. Feeling that power—it's like an incredible orgasm. What an absolute high.

When my wife and I go on vacation, I'm the kind of person who worries about how much we can cram into ten days and whether we'll get to see everything. I make endless lists and itineraries. Riding on the waves, there is no sense of that. I have no thoughts or worries—I just enjoy being there. Before I could bodysurf smoothly, I had to learn a lot about myself—that I could get as much enjoyment out of a small wave as a big wave. I think most people get stuck in the mechanical phase of surfing and spend all of their time thinking about the precise body mechanics or the right wet suit to buy.... I think they forget just to relax and have fun. At one time, I considered riding the small waves as "settling" for them. When the surf wasn't particularly rough on some days, I would be disappointed because I thought that it wouldn't be such an exhilarating or passionate experience. Now I look forward to waves of all sizes and sometimes I take the smaller ones by choice because they are beautiful in a different way. Sexually, there are times I don't even want to get started because I'm afraid I can't finish the "job." Interesting I call it a "job." It keeps me from even wanting to put my foot in the water, so to speak. [Laughs.]

If the wave happens to run out before it gets to the shore, it's really okay. I did the best I could. All waves look good from far away, but when you get to it, the waves sometimes just aren't there. It's okay, though, because I know in my heart there will be another wave. I wish I had the same confidence that there would be another erection if this one "peters out." I just can't believe how many similarities there are between surfing and sex. This is blowing my mind. I never understood sexuality so clearly from the inside before. I really think I understand what you've been saying to me. I need to be comfortable, to not set myself up for failure, to relax and flow with my feelings, and let whatever happens happen—to just enjoy. The size of the wave (or the hardness of my penis) is not the measure of success ... it's the fun ... just the sheer enjoyment of it!

I now realize sexual touching doesn't have to lead to anything ... it is an experience and an end in itself. I guess if I go to the beach and expect there to be waves and they're not there, it's frustrating. But I've learned to enjoy everything about the beach, which is always there even when the waves may not be. This makes me think about what you said about being spontaneous and following what I love during sex. You can never really plan on a wave because it is so out of your control and you can never really force or plan on what will turn you on sexually. But the fun or the potential to enjoy so much with your partner is always there. The parallels have been amazing. I never thought I was good at anything, really. I certainly never thought that my body-surfing would unlock such important awarenesses in me. The joy of surfing has so much to teach me about enjoying sex and the rest of my life. It's just amazing.

Mark came for only two therapy sessions. Later, in a follow-up phone call, he cheerfully reported he was no longer having erection problems. He said, "Everything's great—I'm learning to flow with sex." We're unsure whether he has become supersexual, but he seems to be well on his way.

Rachel, a thirty-six-year-old fitness instructor married for eight years, built an ecstasy connection between sex and her love of dancing. Although she was physically satisfied after sex with her husband Jay, Rachel felt "something was missing" and longed for a deeper connection. "There just has to be more to sex than what I'm feeling," she said. "Sex has become so much like work—so routine—it's almost boring sometimes." Noting that she felt most ecstatic while dancing, Rachel began to build her ecstasy connection to sex.

When I first learned to dance, I was mostly concerned about learning the right steps. I'd watch my feet, but I wasn't focusing on the feeling of the music. Then my dance teacher told me dancing isn't in your feet—it's inside of you. Interesting—I think I'm beginning to see what's happening during sex with Jay. We've bought a number of manuals that teach us different positions (new "steps"), but somehow we've missed the music.

During the next few sessions, Rachel identified her absorption clusters and the mind-set that allowed her to feel so free while dancing. She began to recognize many similarities between the joyous freedom she felt while lost in dance and the sexual ecstasy she could share with Jay.

> When I dance—and it's my song—I just have to get up and move. I feel so free and alive, so much myself, only aware of flowing with the rhythm of the music. When dancing is right, I know it because it feels so effortless and natural. I'm hardly aware of the floor beneath my feet or the other couples on the dance floor. I know that sex can be that effortless: it shouldn't make you tense or worried, it shouldn't be "work," it should be fun. Once you have the "basic" sexual information you can stop worrying about the "steps" and just go with the flow! I can just find that internal rhythm that is mine. I remember trying to follow my friends on the dance floor or copy their style. I learned some of their steps, but my dance teacher told me I would find my own interpretation and it would be right for me. He said I would know it by how it felt, not by how it appeared. I suppose it's learning to pay attention at a different level. Not to break everything down into tinier and tinier parts, but to pay attention to the whole experience. Instead of worrying, "Am I touching Jay the right way?" or whether I'll have an orgasm, I can shift my attention to the whole experience and the sheer pleasure of it all, right?

Rachel was directed to think about what else made dancing so pleasurable. What else did she feel, think about, or imagine while dancing? Her pleasure pattern readily emerged:

> Well, I'm relaxed—very relaxed—but energized at the same time. I feel like I'm really me, having fun without trying. Dancing is a time when I don't hold onto any tension or try to be perfect (like I do in so many other places in my life), I just relax into the music. When I dance, I dance just for me; it's one of the few times I allow myself to be "selfish" that way. My mother died when I was very young and I "took over" for mom, I suppose. Maybe I play the care-

taker role with Jay. It's something to think about. When I
dance, I know it's just me—alone. But when we have sex, I
guess I feel it can't just be for me: I think about Jay a lot
and whether he's okay or having fun. When we have oral
sex, I sometimes worry if I'm doing it right. I would really
have a better time if I focused on my good feelings and
trusted that he'd let me know if he had a problem with what
I was doing; that would really free me to relax. I can see
that I have a choice about whether to take responsibility for
Jay sexually and that my worrying takes something away
from both of us. It sort of robs him of some of his individuality and robs me of my freedom. Letting go of those
worries and paying attention to what I like would be much
better.

I also know that when I dance, there's just a smooth effortless motion, without conscious thought, or so it appears.
My body seems to know what to do without any direction
from my mind. When I dance, I feel like there's an unfold-
ing from the inside. You know what I mean? It's not forced
or phony. This is what I can see myself doing with Jay—I
can really see it! I never thought my passion for dancing
could open up so many ideas about myself that I can apply
to sex. I can't wait to try them. I just hope I can do it!

Worried whether or not she could "do it," Rachel
needed to give herself permission to take the next
step—to avoid striving for some perfect synchronicity or
ideal ecstasy connection and simply allow her body and
feelings to direct her sexual choices. The next time she
had sex with Jay, Rachel approached their lovemaking as if
it were a dance. She focused on the natural rhythms of
their bodies—both her own inner rhythms and the rhythm
of the two of them moving together. By absorbing herself
in the auditory and kinesthetic aspects of lovemaking—the
sounds and movements she loved—she found herself
opening more deeply to sexual pleasure than she ever had.
Rachel was surprised at how simply and beautifully her

love for dance bridged to erotic passion and ecstasy: "I just put on my favorite music, take it into my body the way I do while I'm dancing, and let myself go." When she and Jay were making love, she would imagine sex as gently (or sometimes passionately) moving with her partner across the dance floor, feeling supported in his arms, yet free to improvise and do her own "steps," taking turns leading and following.

Rachel has made some important choices. She chose not to preoccupy herself with notions of touching Jay the "right" way or "working" at sex, but to simply relax into the feeling of pleasure—the way she did while dancing. And what was happening to Jay? He relaxed more, too. As Rachel enjoyed sex more and took responsibility for making it better for herself, Jay let go of his anxieties about worries about Rachel and focused on his enjoyment. Paradoxically, when you and your partner each choose to do what you like, it results in a heightened sexual experience for you both. Rachel and Jay together created their ecstasy connection to supersexual pleasure and beyond.

What is beyond pleasure? It is a truth that is greater than any of our concepts. It is an experience of wholeness, peace, passion and joy; of sexual ecstasy waiting to be savored. It is the possibility of an ultimate connection—a connection with the wonders of the universe. This profound pleasure may come to us abruptly, in one life-changing moment, or gradually over time. It may develop through a change in our focus, actions, feelings, or through a meditative experience. However it comes to you, it will change your thinking forever.

In Closing...and Opening...

We feel so fortunate to have learned about supersex from so many ordinary and yet quite extraordinary women. The women that you have met in this book have been our guides on an exploration of exciting sexual frontiers not well defined or understood before now. Through each of their voices, memories, and images, we have shared in this discovery.

In many ways they are pioneers who have pushed the boundaries of conventional sexual response by describing dimensions and depths of sexual pleasure beyond the "traditional." Their supersexual experiences reflect a connection of mind, body, emotion, and spirit that is the *ultimate* connection, an experience of passion so profound and ineffable that it has defied attempts to package it or attach a precise formula to it. There is no well-worn, familiar path to supersex—each journey is unique.

What we have been introduced to here is a "new" territory for sexual pleasure of our own design—and the boundaries are of our own choosing. As we close ... and open, each of us has the challenge to break new ground and explore endless possibilities that may be lying dormant. Like buried treasure, seemingly lost for years but merely waiting to be unearthed, there is a part of each of us that can be recovered, brought to the surface, where it can be enjoyed because it belongs to each of us.

Becoming more supersexual is something each woman chooses to do for herself. It is an empowering choice that takes us beyond limiting views of the past to the creation of a sexual reality that surpasses expectations. Transcending circumstances, history, and prior beliefs, you learn to trust in yourself and in what you love. In this way, you become the predominant creative force in your own life.

APPENDIX
Guided Imagery

You can record the following guided imagery yourself, or ask someone you trust to read the words into a tape recorder for you. Speak the words in a rhythmic, relaxed tone, as if you were comforting yourself. You may want to record it against some soothing background music. Perhaps you can select music that reminds you of a special time or place. You can choose environmental mood music (sounds of the sea or woodland) or a favorite evocative piece. As you read emphasized words, modify your tone. For example, as you read the word *deep,* lower your voice and slow it down a bit. If the word *peaceful* is emphasized, read the word with a peaceful inflection. When you see a number of dots in succession, this indicates a pause. Take some time to pause and leave some quiet space on the tape. Depending upon your preference, this can be from ten seconds to thirty seconds or longer. During the pauses, allow yourself to gently focus on your breathing and any feelings of relaxation or pleasantness. As you prac-

221

tice, you will discover how long a pause to include for you
to experience the images fully and vividly. In time, you will
find the right music, voice, and pacing to help you relax,
enjoy the images that emerge, and quiet your mind. Remember, there is no right or wrong way to enjoy this
guided imagery. Whatever works for you is right.

Getting as physically comfortable as you possibly can—
and just letting your mind become clear of any thoughts or
distractions or worries . . . allowing your conscious mind to
relax as your unconscious mind begins to cultivate some
very positive imagery . . . and you can simply watch what
is happening as if you are witnessing an inner drama—as
if you were seeing it on a movie screen that rolls behind
your eyelids—and to promote that imagery, just let yourself relax as completely as you can . . . wherever you happen to find yourself, whether you're lying down or sitting
in a chair—just let yourself sink *comfortably* into that spot
. . . and feel free to move around to get as comfortable as
you possibly can . . . taking several deep breaths to assist
in the process of relaxation (pause), each breath having
that pleasantness about it that encourages a very *deep* relaxation, that's what you're going for, *depth* . . . (pause) to
the point where you can create within your own self that
wonderful feeling of heaviness, so that your arms, your
hands, and your fingers feel *heavy,* make them feel heavy,
make your legs feel heavy . . . feel the pull of gravity . . .
that mysterious force . . . *feel it* . . . notice how some parts
of your body can feel that pull of gravity more than others,
feel that pull of gravity drawing you gently but firmly
deeper and deeper into the place where you are . . . letting
that pleasant heaviness, that relaxation, *spread* throughout
your body . . . and there is no right or wrong depth of
relaxation—your unconscious mind can make choices
about how deeply you will go into relaxation—and how will

you know when you are deeply relaxed?—maybe your muscles will change in some way—or just the sensation of letting go to the calmness and serenity of the moment—as if the rest of world disappears—letting any distractions simply come and go—beginning to focus on a very positive image and allow yourself to immerse yourself in the experience—as if the experience were a river and the river represents time—so you wade into time and are immersed in present or past or coming into future—time flows—smell a familiar smell and instantly you are in childhood—or a familiar cologne and you are in your lover's arms—or a certain song you haven't heard for years—you may begin to notice a certain change in the flow of time or a sense of detachment—as you become more in tune with your experiences—opening to the possibilities of limitless pleasure and boundless joy—moving to wherever your journey takes you—trusting that you know joy because your unconscious mind is an expert in joy—and taking comfort in knowing that there is something more that you can feel and experience—something you *can* have—naturally—comfortably ... rhythmically following your breathing as you take in pleasurable energy with each inhale and with each breath out—letting go of all the tension—or pressure—or strain—things you really don't need (pause)—It feels so good to take a moment for yourself—so effortlessly—so comfortably. Learning about your inner wisdom—

And—when you are ready—in your mind's eye—with the kind of clarity you happen to be capable of at this time, create a scene, perhaps a walk in a park—beautiful blue sky, trees that are colorful ... leaves alive with fall colors—the reds, the oranges, the greens ... some leaves perhaps already on the ground adding a touch of reddish orange ... green grass still there so you get the contrast ... perhaps a body of water such as a pond and the pond is smooth as glass and reflective so that you can see the trees with their mirror image on the water . . . and perhaps a few leaves already floating on the water as well . . . how interesting it is to take a small stone or pebble and just toss it in the water and hear the *blup* and to watch the concentric rings that are produced . . . watch those rings— how fascinating—as they spread out (pause), and from one very small circle they get *bigger* and *bigger* and *bigger* and from one little ring, there are many many rings gently expanding across the surface of the water . . . it's so beautifully peaceful . . . the air is fresh and clean . . . it has that fall fragrance, tune into that freshness, that fall fragrance . . . letting yourself go *deeper* and *deeper* and *deeper* into pleasantness . . . into *calm* . . . quietly pleasant . . . quietly calm . . . perhaps the sound of a bird . . . singing . . . that sense of being one with nature . . . the simple beauty, the marvelous complexity . . . seeing that scene through poetic eyes, through the eyes of an artist . . . tune in to the warmth of the sun and the coolness of the air . . . to the sound of the leaves as you walk along . . . the sound of those leaves crunching underfoot . . . tune in to the peacefulness, that *wonderful* peacefulness . . . your mind focusing on nature in all its magnificence . . . and feeling that *oneness,* that communion with nature . . . that oneness with the universe . . . the substance of your being is the substance of the universe, you share a unity there . . . experience that unity, that oneness, the comfort, the power, the peacefulness (pause) . . . let yourself go *deep* into the pleasure . . . tuning into all that your mind can grasp . . . that wonderful beauty . . . the marvel of a leaf as it falls from a tree, *gently,* it glides on the air . . . and it comes to rest so delicately . . . it glistens in the sunlight to the point of iridescence . . . and you can feel one with that leaf . . . appreciating its beauty . . . it's so simple and yet it's so complex . . . it's so finite and yet it's so infinite . . . the water . . . so peaceful ... the pond itself is fed by a brook ... and the brook meanders through a field ... a grassy field, the brook itself has rocks and stones, so as the water passes over it—it burbles and gurgles at certain points ... the water is clear and clean and fresh and cool ... a delight just to stoop down and press some against your face and feel its freshness, its coolness ... *letting yourself relax even more deeply* ... sharing ... with nature ... appreciating the unity you have with nature ... and having the freedom to become everything that you see ... to appreciate the tree by becoming the tree and to appreciate the brook by becoming the brook ... or becoming the pond ... or the sky ... or the clouds or the sun or the fresh air ... appreciating that everything that exists is composed of the same basic matter, it's just that things are organized differently ... there's a kind of poetry in that ... let that poetic dimension draw you even *deeper* ... eliciting from yourself a very positive response ... feeling the energy fill your being ... it's as if you've suddenly become plugged into the universe itself and you're becoming charged up with the power and the force of the universe ... it creates within you a source of well-being, a feeling of comfort, and an appreciation of yourself ... yourself as a woman ... an appreciation of your value and your worth, an appreciation of sharing ... sharing with the universe ... sharing with nature ... the magnificent harmony and order of the universe is within yourself ... and that produces such profound *peace* ... *let yourself go deeper* ... letting go of any distractions ... and just letting yourself comfortably relax—just letting the experience be totally part of yourself (pause) ... the energy ... the vitality ... producing such a wonderful feeling within yourself ... the use of your fantasy ... the wondrous effortless wisdom of your inner voice—listen to it—learning of a new vision—a new clarity—a power—and the more you tune into that wisdom, letting yourself go *deep* into pleasure, the more complete you are ... the stronger you are ... the more at peace you are ... the relaxation has a wonderful influence over your entire being ... you are strengthened in a marvelous way ... discovering a wisdom just waiting to be enjoyed—going on a deeper feeling level ... comfortably *relaxed* ... feeling so *wonderful* ... an uplifting sense rises within you ... it's the feeling of well-being associated with being in a wonderful place ... and the experience is one that is new and different each time ... no two scenes are exactly alike and yet the experience produces such peace ... you feel totally yourself ... you don't have to do anything special ... being yourself is sufficient ... you *can* let go of all of those things from the past that influence you in a negative way and you *can* let yourself learn and grow—tune in to the power and the energy that is always there ... so that without even thinking you find yourself uplifted and strengthened ... thinking and feeling very creatively and positively ... recognizing the pleasure centers and feeling them within yourself or with your lover—feeling free to discover new sensory awareness—excitement and sexual joy—(pause) ... feeling a oneness within yourself ... feeling a soundness and a wholeness ... body and mind become completely synchronized and the harmony flows so smoothly ... that wonderful feeling of peace ... tune in to it within yourself—it's there and it grows ... that *feeling beyond pleasure—*

And each time you listen to this guided imagery—you will find yourself going even more deeply and easily into pleasure and calm—discovering infinite possibilities for ecstasy—and—whenever you wish—at your own pace—slowly bring yourself back—feeling calm and relaxed and much better than before.

BIBLIOGRAPHY

This book has been written for the general reader, however, scientists and curious laypeople may well want to do follow-up reading and research on a number of provocative points. For these readers, we have provided this full bibliography of all resources used throughout the years of scientific investigation on which this book is based.

Abramson, P.R. "The relationship of the frequency of masturbation to several aspects of personality and behavior." *Journal of Sex Research* 9 2, (1973): 132–42.

Abramson, P.R. and D.L. Mosher. "Development of a measure of negative attitudes toward masturbation." *Journal of Clinical and Consulting Psychology* 43 (1975): 485–90.

Abramson, P.R. and D.L. Mosher. "An empirical investigation of experimentally induced masturbatory fantasies." *Archives of Sexual Behavior* 8 1 (1979): 27–39.

Adams, A.E., S.N. Haynes, and M.A. Brayer. "Cognitive distraction in female sexual arousal." *Psychophysiology 22* 6 (1985): 689–96.

Adams, C.L. "An informal preliminary report on some factors relating to sexual responsiveness of certain college wives." In M.F. DeMartino (ed.), *Sexual Behavior and Personality Characteristics.* New York: Citadel, 1963.

Ahsen, A. "Eidetics: An overview." *Journal of Mental Imagery* 1 (1979): 5–38.

American Psychological Association. *Ethical Principles in the Conduct of Research with Human Participants.* Washington, D.C., 1982.

Anand, M. *The Art of Sexual Ecstasy.* Los Angeles, California; Jeremy P. Tarcher, Inc, 1989.

Anderson, J. "Arguments concering representations for mental imagery." *Psychological Review* 85 (1978): 249–78.

Anderson, M.P. "Imaginal processes: Therapeutic applications and theoretical models." In M.J. Mahoney (ed.), *Psychotherapy Process: Current Issues and Future Directions.* New York: Plenum, 1980, pp. 211–48.

Annon, J.S. *Behavioral Treatment of Sexual Problems.* New York: Harper & Row, 1976.

As, A., J.W. O'Hara, and M.P. Munger. "The measurement of subjective experiences presumably related to hypnotic susceptibility." *Scandinavian Journal of Psychology* 3 (1962): 47–64.

Austin, C.R. and R.V. Short. *Human Sexuality.* Cambridge: Cambridge University Press, 1980.

Bandler, R. and J. Grinder. *Patterns of the Hypnotic Techniques of Milton H. Erickson, M.D.* (Vol. 1). Cupertino, California: Meta Publications, 1975.

Bandler, R. and J. Grinder. *Frogs into Princes.* Moab, Utah: Real People Press, 1979.

Barbach, Lonnie. *Erotic Interludes.* New York: HarperCollins, 1987.

Barbach, Lonnie. *For Yourself.* New York: Signet, 1976.

Barber, T.X. and L.B. Glass. "Significant factors in hypnotic behavior." *Journal of Abnormal and Social Psychology* 69 (1962): 222–28.

Beck, A.T. *Cognitive Therapy and the Emotional Disorders.* New York: International Universities Press, 1976.

Benson, H. *The Relaxation Response.* New York: Avon Books, 1976.

Buber, M. *I and Thou.* New York: Scribners, 1958.

Bucke, R.M. *Cosmic Consciousness.* New York: E.P. Dutton, 1923.

Byrne, D. and L. Byrne (eds). *Exploring Human Sexuality.* New York: Crowell, 1977.

Campbell, J. *Myths to Live By.* New York: Viking Penguin, 1972.

Campbell, J. with B. Moyers. *The Power of Myth.* New York: Doubleday, 1988.

Carson, R.C. "Self-fulfilling prophecy, maladaptive behavior, and psychotherapy." In J.C. Anchin and D.J. Kiesler (eds)., *Handbook of Interpersonal Psychotherapy,* New York: Pergamon, 1982, pp. 64–77.

Cautela, J.R. "Covert sensitization." *Psychological Record 20* (1967): 459–68.

Crawford, H.J. "Hypnotizability, daydreaming styles, imagery vividness, and absorption: A multidimensional study." *Journal of Personality and Social Psychology 42* 5 (1982): 915–26.

Csikszentmihalyi, M. and I.S. Csikszentmihalyi. *Optimal Experience.* Cambridge: Cambridge University Press, 1988.

Csikszentmihalyi, M. *Flow: The Psychology of Optimal Experience.* New York: Harper & Row, 1990.

Davidson, J.K. and L.E. Hoffman. "Sexual fantasies and sexual satisfaction: an empirical analysis of erotic thought." *Journal of Sex Research 22* 2 (1986): 184–205.

Deutsch, H. *The Psychology of Women.* New York: Grune & Stratton, 1944.

Ellis, A. "An impolite interview with Albert Ellis." *Monograph of the Institute for Rational Living,* New York, 1960.

Ellis, A. *Reason and Emotion.* New York: Stuart Books, 1962.

Erikson, M.H., E.L. Rossi, and R. Rossi. *Hypnotic Realities: The Induction of Clinical Hypnosis and Forms of Indirect Suggestion.* New York: Irvington Publishers, Inc., 1976.

Feuerstein, G. *Sacred Sexuality.* Los Angeles: J.P. Tarcher, 1992.

Fisher, S. *The Female Orgasm.* New York: Basic Books, 1973.

Flowers, J.V. and C.D. Boorham. "Imagination training in the treatment of sexual dysfunction." *Counseling Psychologist* 5 (1975): 50–51.

Frankl, V.E. *Man's Search for Meaning.* New York: Pocket Books, 1963.

Freedman, R. *Bodylove.* New York: Harper & Row, Publishers, 1988.

Freud, S. "Three essays on the theory of sexuality." In J. Strachey (ed. and trans.), *Standard Edition of the Complete Psychological Works of Sigmund Freud.* London: Hogarth Press, 1953 (original work published 1905), pp. 123–245.

Freud, S. "Hysterical phantasies and bisexuality." In J. Strachey (ed. and trans.), *Standard Edition of the Complete Psychological Works of Sigmund Freud.* London: Hogarth Press, 1953 (original work published 1908), pp. 51–58.

Fromm, E. *To Have or To Be?* New York: Harper & Row, 1976.

Gagnon, J.H. and W. Simon. *Sexual Conduct.* Chicago: Aldine Press, 1973.

Gallwey, T., and B. Kriegel. *Inner Skiing.* New York: Bantam Books, 1977.

Garfield, C. A. *Peak Peformance.* New York: Warner Books, 1984.

Green, S.E. and D.L. Mosher. "A causal model of sexual arousal to erotic fantasies." *Journal of Sex Research* 21 (1985): 1–22.

Greenberg, L.S. and J.D. Safran. *Emotion in Psychotherapy: Affect, Cognition, and the Process of Change.* New York: Guilford, 1987.

Hanh, T. N. *The Miracle of Mindfulness! A Manual on Meditation.* Boston: Beacon Press, 1976.

Hariton, E.B. and J.L. Singer. "Women's fantasies during sexual intercourse." *Journal of Consulting and Clinical Psychology* 42 (1974): 313–22.

Harrell, T.H. and R.D. Stolp. "Effects of erotic guided imagery on female sexual arousal and emotional response." *Journal of Sex Research* 21 (1985): 292–304.

Harris, H., S. Yulis, and D. LaCoste. "Relationships among sexual arousability, imagery ability and introversion-extraversion." *Journal of Sex Research* 16 (1980): 72–86.

Heiman, J.R. "A psychophysiological explanation of sexual

arousal patterns in females and males." *Psychophysiology* 14 (1977): 266–74.

Heiman, J.R. "Uses of psychophysiology in the assessment and treatment of sexual dysfunction." In J. LoPiccolo and L. LoPiccolo (eds.), *Handbook of Sex Therapy*, 1978, New York: Plenum, pp. 123–35.

Heiman, J.R. and J. Hatch. "Conceptual and therapeutic contributions of psychophysiology to sexual dysfunctions." In S.N. Haynes and L.R. Gannon (eds.), *Psychophysiological Approach to Etiology and Treatment*. New York: Praeger, 1981.

Heimer, J.R., L. LoPiccolo, and J. LoPiccolo. *Becoming Orgasmic: A Sexual Growth Program for Women*. Englewood Cliffs, New Jersey: Prentice-Hall, 1976.

Heyn, D. *The Erotic Silence of the American Wife*. New York: Random House, 1992.

Hite, S. *The Hite Report: A Nationwide Study of Female Sexuality*. New York: Dell, 1976.

Hollender, M.H. "Women's fantasies during sexual intercourse." *Archives of General Psychiatry* 8 (1963): 86–90.

Hoon, P.W., J.P. Wincze, and E.F. Hoon. "The effect of biofeedback and cognitive mediation upon vaginal blood volume." *Behavior Therapy* 8 (1977): 694–702.

Horowitz, H.J. *Image Formation and Psychotherapy*. New York: Jason Aronson, 1983.

Hoyt, I.P., et al. "Daydreaming, absorption and hypnotizability." *International Journal of Clinical and Experimental Hypnosis* *37* 4 (1989): 332–42.

Jung, C.G. *The Archetypes and the Collective Unconscious*. New York: Pantheon, 1959.

Kaats, G.R. and K.E. Davis. "Effects of volunteer biases in studies of sexual behavior and attitudes." *Journal of Sex Research* 7 (1971): 513–20.

Kabat-Zinn, J. *Full Catastrophe Living*. New York: Delacorte, 1990.

Kaplan, H.S. *The New Sex Therapy: Active Treatment of Sexual Dysfunctions*. New York: Brunner/Mazel, 1974.

Kelly, L.A.S. "Imagining ability, marital adjustment and erotic fantasy during sexual relations in married men and wom-

232 Bibliography

en." *Dissertations Abstracts International 39,* 1457B–1458B
(University Microfilms No. 78-15, 595), 1978.

Korzybski, A. *Science and Sanity: An Introduction to Non-
Aristotelian Systems and General Semantics.* Lancaster, PA:
Science Press, 1933.

Krishnamurti, J. *Commentaries on Living.* Wheaton, Illinois: The
Theosophical Publishing House, 1986.

Kumar, V.K. and R.J. Pekala. "Hypnotizability, absorption, and individual difference in phenomenological experience." *International Journal of Clinical and Experimental Hypnosis 36* 2
(1988): 80–88.

Lang, P.J. "A bio-informational theory of emotional imagery."
Psychophysiology 16 (1979): 495–512.

Lazarus, A.A. *The Practice of Multimodal Therapy.* New York:
McGraw-Hill, 1981.

Leonard, George. *The Silent Pulse.* New York: E.P. Dutton, 1978.

Leuner, H. "Guided affective imagery (GAI): A method of inten-
sive psychotherapy." *American Journal of Psychotherapy 34* 4
(1969).

Lobitz, W.C. and J. LoPiccolo. "New methods in the behavioral
treatment of sexual dysfunction." *Journal of Behavioral and
Experimental Psychiatry* 3 (1972): 265–71.

Lynn, S.J. and J.W. Rhue. "The fantasy-prone person: hypnosis,
imagination and creativity." *Journal of Personality and Social
Psychology 51* 2 (1986): 404–8.

Mahoney, M.J. *Cognition and Behavior Modification.* Cambridge,
Massachusetts: Ballinger Press, 1974.

Mandler, G. *Mind and Emotion.* New York: John Wiley, 1972.

Mann, J. "Experimental induction of sexual arousal." *Technical
Report of the Commission on Obscenity and Pornography.*
Washington, D.C.: U.S. Government Printing Office, Vol. 1
(1971): pp. 23–61.

Maslow, A.H. "Self-esteem and sexuality in women." *Journal of
Social Psychology* 16 (1942): 259–64.

Maslow, A.H. *The Farther Reaches of Human Nature.* New York:
Viking Penguin, 1971.

Masters, W.H. and V.E. Johnson. *Human Sexual Inadequacy.*
Boston: Little, Brown, 1970.

Meichenbaum, D. *Cognitive-Behavior Modification.* New York: Plenum, 1977.

Mischel, W. "Personality and cognition: something borrowed, something new." In N. Cantor and J.F. Kihlstrom (eds.), *Personality, Cognition and Social Interaction.* Hillsdale, New Jersey: Erlbaum, 1981, pp. 3–19.

Money, J. *Lovemaps.* New York: Irvington Publishers, Inc. 1976.

Morokoff, P.J. "Volunteer bias in the psychophysiological study of female sexuality." *Journal of Sex Research 22* 1 (1986): 35–51.

Mosher, D.L. "Three dimensions of depth of involvement in human sexual response." *Journal of Sex Research* 16 (1980): 1–42.

Mosher, D.L. and P.R. Abramson. "Subjective sexual arousal to films of masturbation." *Journal of Consulting and Clinical Psychology* 45 (1977): 796–807.

Mosher, D.L. and B.B. White. "Effects of committed or casual erotic guided imagery on female subjective sexual arousal and emotional response." *Journal of Sex Research 16* 4 (1980): 273–99.

Mosher, D.L., M.A. Barton-Henry, and S.E. Green. *The Measurement of Subjective Sexual Arousal.* Unpublished manuscript, 1984.

Neisser, U. *Cognitive Psychology.* New York: Appleton-Century-Crofts, 1967.

Neisser, U. *Cognition and Reality.* San Francisco: W.H. Freeman, 1976.

Neisser, U. "Anticipations, images and introspection." *Cognition* 6 (1978): 169–74.

Nutter, D.E. and M.K. Condron. "Sexual fantasy and activity patterns of females with inhibited sexual desire vs. normal controls." *Journal of Sex and Marital Therapy 9* 4 (1983): 276–82.

Paivio, A. "Perceptual comparisons through the mind's eye." *Memory and Cognition* 3 (1975): 635–47.

Paivio, A. *Mental Representations: A Dual Coding Approach.* New York: Oxford University Press, 1986.

Palmer, R.D. and P.B. Field. "Visual imagery and susceptibility to hypnosis." *Journal of Consulting and Clinical Psychology* *32* 4 (1968): 456–61.

Peck, M. S. *The Road Less Traveled.* New York: Simon & Schuster, 1978.

Pekala, R.J., C.F. Wenger, and R.L. Levine. "Individual differences in phenomenological experience: States of consciousness as a function of absorption." *Journal of Personality and Social Psychology 48* 1 (1985): 125–32.

Perry, C. "Imagery, fantasy, and hypnotic susceptibility: A multidimensional approach." *Journal of Personality and Social Psychology 24* 2 (1973): 217–21.

Piaget, J. and B. Inhelder. *Memory and Intelligence.* New York: Basic Books, 1973.

Plutchick, R. *Emotion.* New York: Academic Press, 1980.

Posner, M.I. "Cumulative development of attentional theory." *American Psychologist 37* (1982): 168–79.

Privette, G. "Peak experience, peak performance and flow: A comparative analysis of positive human experience." *Journal of Personality and Social Psychology 83* 45 (1983): 1361–68.

Pryzbyla, D.P.J., D. Byrne, and K. Kelley. "The role of imagery in sexual behavior." In A.A. Sheikh (ed.), *Imagery: Current Theory, Resarch and Application.* New York: John Wiley, 1983, pp. 436–67.

Pylyshyn, Z.W. "What the mind's eye tells the mind's brain: A critique of mental imagery." *Psychological Bulletin 80* 1 (1973): 1–24.

Qualls, P.J. and P.W. Sheehan. "Capacity for absorption and relaxation during electromyograph biofeedback and no-feedback conditions." *Journal of Abnormal Psychology 88* 6 (1979): 652–62.

Reich, W. *The Discovery of the Orgone: The Function of the Orgasm.* New York: Noonday, 1942.

Reyner, J. "Free imagery: An uncovering procedure." *Journal of Clinical Psychology 19* (1963): 454.

Richardson, A. "Imagery: definition and types." In A.A. Sheikh (ed.), *Imagery: Current Theory, Research and Application.* New York: John Wiley, 1983, pp. 3–42.

Roberts, C.R. *Depth of Involvement, Imagery, and Daydreaming: A Study of Altered States of Consciousness and Orgasmic Suc-*

cess in Women. Ann Arbor, Michigan: University Microfilms International, 1983.

Roche, S.M., and K.M. McConkey. "Absorption: Nature, assessment and correlates." *Journal of Personality and Social Psychology,* 59 (1990): 91–101.

Rosenthal, R. and R. Rosnow. "The volunteer subject." In R. Rosenthal and R.L. Rosnow (eds.), *Artifact in Behavioral Research.* New York: Academic Press, 1969, pp. 59–118.

Safron, J.D. and L.S. Greenberg. "Cognitive appraisal and reappraisal: implications for clinical practice." *Cognitive Therapy and Research* 6 (1982a): 252–58.

Safron, J.D. and L.S. Greenberg. "Eliciting hot cognitions in cognitive behavior therapy: rationale and procedural guidelines." *Canadian Psychology* 23 (1982b): 83–87.

Scantling, S.R. "The relationships among attitudes toward sexual fantasy, depth of absorption, and subjective sexual arousal in women: The experimental use of guided imagery." Unpublished doctoral dissertation, Antioch/New England Graduate School, 1990.

Schnarch, D.M. *Constructing the Sexual Crucible.* New York: W.W. Norton, 1991.

Schultz, W.C. *Joy: Twenty Years Later.* Berkeley, California: Ten Speed Press, 1989.

Shainess, N. and H. Greenwald. "Debate: Are fantasies during sexual relations a sign of difficulty?" *Sexual Behavior 1 2* (1971): 38–54.

Sheehan, P.W. "Reliability of a short test of imagery." *Perceptual and Motor Skills* 25 (1967): 744.

Sheehan, P.W. "Hypnosis and the process of imagination." In E. Fromm and R.E. Shor (eds.), *Hypnosis: Developments in Research and New Perspectives.* New York: Aldine, 1979.

Shevrin, H. and S. Dickman. "The psychological unconscious: A necessary assumption for all psychological theory?" *American Psychologist* 35 (1980): 421–34.

Shor, R.E., M.T. Orne, and D.N. O'Connell. "Validation and cross-validation of a scale of self-reported personal experiences which predict hypnotizability." *Journal of Psychology* 53 (1962): 55–75.

Siegel, Bernie S. *Love, Medicine and Miracles.* New York: Harper & Row, 1986.

Sinetar, M. *Ordinary People as Monks and Mystics.* New York: Paulist Press, 1986.

Singer, B. "Conceptualizing sexual arousal and attraction." *Journal of Sex Research 20* 3 (1984): 230–40.

Singer, J.L. *Imagery and Daydream Methods in Psychotherapy and Behavior Modification.* New York: Academic Press., 1974.

Sirkin, M.I. *Sexual Involvement Theory, Sexual Trance, and Hypnotizability: The Experimental Use of Guided Imagery.* Unpublished doctoral dissertation, University of Connecticut, 1985.

Spencer, H. *The Principles of Psychology,* Vol. 1. New York: Appleton, 1890.

Stampfl, T.G. and D.J. Levis. "Essentials of implosive therapy." *Journal of Abnormal Psychology* 72 (1967): 496–503.

Stevens, B. *Don't Push the River.* Berkeley, California: Celestial Arts, 1970.

Stock, W.E. and J.H. Geer. "A study of fantasy-based sexual arousal in women." *Archives of Sexual Behavior 11* 1 (1982): 33–47.

Sue, D. "Erotic fantasies of college students during coitus." *Journal of Sex Research* 15 (1979): 299–305.

Tellegen, A. and G. Atkinson. "Openness to absorbing and self-altering experiences ('Absorption'), a trait related to hypnotic susceptibility." *Journal of Abnormal Psychology* 83 (1974): 268–77.

Tellegen, A. "Practicing the two disciplines for relaxation and enlightment: Comment on Qualls and Sheehan." *Journal of Experimental Psychology: General, 110* (1981): 217–226.

Tellegen, A. *Brief Manual for the Multidimensional Personality Questionnaire.* Unpublished manuscript, University of Minnesota, Minneapolis, 1982.

Tellegen, A. *"Discussion: Hypnosis and Absorption."* Paper presented at the 38th annual meeting of the Society for Clinical and Experimental Hypnosis, Los Angeles, California, October, 1987.

Tellegen, A. *"A new 'element-centered' nonmetric scaling method (Escal)."* Unpublished manuscript. University of Minnesota, Minneapolis, 1992.

Tellegen, A. and N.G. Waller. (in press). "Exploring personality through test construction: Development of the Multidimensional Personality Questionnaire." In S. R. Briggs & J. M. Cheek (eds.), *Personality Measures: Development and Evaluation* (vol. 1). Greenwich, Connecticut: JAI Press.

Thomas, L. *The Lives of a Cell.* New York: Viking, 1974.

Walen, S.R. "Cognitive factors in sexual behavior." *Journal of Sex and Marital Therapy* 6 2 (1980): 87–101.

Whalen, R.E. "Sexual motivation." *Psychological Review* 73 (1966): 151–63.

Wilbur, K. *No Boundary.* Boston: New Science Library, 1981.

Wilson, S.C. and T.X. Barber. "Vivid fantasy and hallucinatory abilities in the life histories of excellent hypnotic subjects ('Somnambules'): Preliminary report with female subjects." In E. Klinger (ed.), *Imagery: Concepts, Results and Applications.* New York: Plenum, 1981, pp. 133–49.

Wilson, S.C. and T.X. Barber. "The fantasy-prone personality: Implications for understanding imagery, hypnosis, and parapsychological phenomena." In A.A. Sheikh (ed.), *Imagery: Current Theory, Research and Application.* New York: John Wiley, 1983, pp. 340–90.

Winnicott, D.W. *Mother and Child.* New York: Basic Books, 1957.

Wolchik, S.A., S.L. Braver, and K. Jensen. "Volunteer bias in erotica research: Effects of intrusiveness of measure and sexual background." *Archives of Sexual Behavior* 14 (1985): 93–107.

Wolchik, S.A., S.L. Spencer, and I.S. Lisi. "Volunteer bias in research employing vaginal measures of sexual arousal: Demographic, sexual and personality characteristics." *Archives of Sexual Behavior* 12 (1983): 399–408.

Wolpe, J. *The Practice of Behavior Therapy.* New York: Pergamon, 1974.

Yuille, J.C. and M.J. Catchpole. "The role of imagery in models of cognition." *Journal of Mental Imagery* 1 (1977): 171–80.

Zuckerman, M. "Physiological measures of sexual arousal in humans." In N.S. Greenfield and R.A. Sternbach (eds.), *Handbook of Psychophysiology.* New York: Holt, Rinehart & Winston, 1972, pp. 709–40.

Zukav, Gary. *The Dancing Wu Li Masters.* New York: Bantam, 1979.

Authors' Note:
Notes on Structure of the MPQ Absorption Scale

The seven clusters of absorption presented in *Ordinary Women, Extraordinary Sex* utilized Auke Tellegen's earlier research (1981) as a guide. The clusters have been modified and applied to supersexual experience based on our clinical findings. Dr. Tellegen's most recent factor analyses of these clusters (Tellegen & Waller, in press) presents a six-factor matrix of correlations taken from a sample of 2000. Based on this analysis, Tellegen concludes, "Absorption appears to represent a disposition to enter (under conducive circumstances) psychological states that are characterized by marked restructuring of the phenomenal self and world ... that may have a peak-experience-like quality. They may have an external focus, or may reflect an inner focus on reminiscences, images, and imaginings. The absorption trait subsumes these diverse possibilities in a remarkable cohesive correlational structure." He further states that each of these factors is highly intercorrelated (Note on Structure and Meaning of The MPQ Scale, Tellegen, 1992).

This provides convincing statistical evidence that absorption is a phenomenon composed of many interconnected facets and although we have discussed the clusters of absorption separately, they are part of a unified whole.

Index

Absorbers
  high, 141, 180–183, 198
  low, 141, 150–157
  medium, 141, 150–151,
    157–180
  See also Absorption
Absorption
  clusters to, 141–150
  as critical to supersex, 136
  as dimension of peak
    experience, 61–62
  spectrum of, 136–137,
    150–151
  term defined, 135–136
  See also Absorbers
Abuse, and disassociation,
    100–101
Acceptance, feeling of,
    supersex and, 81,
    83–84
Ackerman, Diane, 199–200

Actual Minds, Possible Worlds
  (Bruner), 114
Age, as nonfactor in supersex,
    107–108
Aliveness, intense, as
  dimension of peak
  experience, 62
Altered state of consciousness
  orgasm and, 24–25
  supersex and, 24–25
Anand, Margo, 29–30
Archives of Sexual Behavior,
  27
Arousal, and sexual fantasies,
    201–202
Art of Sexual Ecstasy, The
  (Anand), 29
Association for Humanistic
  Psychology, 64–65
"At home," feeling of,
  supersex and, 51–52

241

Balance, feeling of, supersex
  and, 128–132, 137
Beginner's mind, cultivating,
  as facet of supersexual
  mind-set, 186, 196–200
Benson, Herbert, 188
Bernstein, Leonard, 60–61
Bodylove (Freedman), 83
Bruner, Jerome, 114
Buber, Martin, 63, 74–76, 129
Buddha, 119, 129, 187
Buddhism, mysticism and sex
  in, 24–25
Byers, Dr. Paul, 64, 65

Campbell, Joseph, 47–48, 52
Certainty, suspending, as
  facet of supersexual
  mind-set, 186, 196–200
Charisma, as characteristic of
  supersexual woman,
  103–104
Chinen, Allen B., 114
Clusters to absorption,
  141–150
Colors, as manifestation of
  supersexual ecstasy, 7,
  19, 28, 29, 34–35, 40,
  148
Commitment, supersex and,
  80, 81
Communication
  lack of, as problem in
    unsatisfying sex, 8
  satisfying sex, 8
  Supersex and, 52
Concentration, relaxed,
  supersex and, 50

Connectedness, sense of,
  supersex and, 64–67
Connection
  ecstasy, building, 207, 209
  spiritual (Cluster 7),
    149–150
Consciousness, altered state
  of
  and orgasm, 24–25
  supersex and, 24–25
Control, and letting go
  effect of, on supersexual
    women, 119–120
  supersex and, 129, 137
Courage, as characteristic of
  supersexual women,
    93–94, 98, 102
Cross-sensory experience
  (Cluster 6), 148
Csikszentmihalyi, Mihalyi,
  59–61

Dancing Wu Li Masters, The
  (Zukav), 63
Davidson, Julian M., 24–25
Daydreaming
  effect of, on supersexual
    women, 115–116
  and fantasy (Cluster 5), 147
Desire, lack of, and
  unsatisfying sex, 8
Disassociation
  and abuse, 100–101
  and sexuality, 100
Distraction, tuning out
  (Cluster 1), 143
Divorce, post-, supersex,
  40–43

Drama of the Gifted Child (Miller), 193

Ecstasy
connection, building, 207, 209
supersexual
as learned experience, 14
manifestations of, 6–7, 19–20, 28–30, 40
Ecstasy: A Study of Some Secular and Religious Experiences (Laski), 20
Ecstasy: A Way of Knowing (Greeley), 21
Einstein, Albert, 66
Emotions, feeling, in response to "external" cues (Clusters 2 and 3), 143–144
Endowments, physical, importance of, as myth of satisfactory sex, 17
Entrainment, term defined, 65
Erotic Silence of the American Wife, The (Heyn), 29
Experience(s)
cross-sensory (Cluster 6), 148
life-threatening, and sudden supersexual transformation, 128
peak. *See* Peak experience

Fairy Tales
effect of, on supersexual women, 113–115
See also Fantasy
Fear of Flying (Jong), 73

Fantasy(ies)
daydreaming and (Cluster 5), 147
effect of, on supersexual women, 113–116
enhancing enjoyment of, as facet of supersexual mind-set, 186, 200–207
sexual, arousal and, 201–202
Feuerstein, Georg, Ph.D., 28
Flow, supersex and, 59–61, 121
For Whom the Bell Tolls (Hemingway), 31–32
Frankl, Viktor, 99–100
Freedman, Rita, 83
Fromm, Erich, 48–49
Full Catastrophe Living (Kabat-Zinn), 66

Geer, James H., 116
Gestalt psychology, 50
Greeley, Andrew M., 21, 22, 23

Harmony, sense of, supersex and, 128–132
Hemingway, Ernest, 31–32
Heyn, Dalma, 28–29
"High Sex," 29
Hinduism, Tantric, mysticism and sex in, 24–25, 30
Hite, Shere, 25–26
Hite Report (Hite), 26
Honesty, as characteristic of supersexual woman, 97–98
Horney, Karen, 94

Human Sexual Response
    (Masters and
    Johnson), 25
Huygens, Christiaan, 65

I-It relationships, 75
Image, term defined, 201
Images, enhancing enjoyment
    of, as facet of
    supersexual mind-set,
    186, 200–207
Independence, as
    characteristic of
    supersexual women,
    103
Insight, sudden, effect of, on
    supersexual women,
    117–119
Intercourse, first, as
    disappointing
    experience, 14–16
I-Thou relationships, 74–77,
    149

James, William, 7–8
Jesus, 129
Jong, Erica, 73
Joy, supersexual. *See* Ecstasy,
    supersexual
Jung, Carl, 63, 101, 129

Kabat-Zinn, Dr. Jon, 66–67
"Knowing," sense of,
    supersex and, 52–54
Korzybski, Alfred, 55

Language of the Senses, The
    (Ackerman), 199
Laski, Margharita, 20–21, 23

Leonard, George, 56–57,
    64–65, 103
Letting go
    control and
    supersex and, 137
    effect of, on supersexual
    women, 119–120
    feeling of, supersex and, 56
Letting moment lead, as facet
    of supersexual mind-
    set, 186, 188–190
Lewis, C. S., 128
Lord of the Flies (Golding),
    114
Lord of the Rings, The
    (Tolkien), 113

Man's Search for Meaning
    (Frankl), 99
Maslow, Abraham, 23–24,
    61–62
Masters and Johnson, sex
    studies of, 25
Meditation, supersex and,
    187–188
Miller, Alice, 193
Mind
    beginner's, cultivating, as
    facet of supersexual
    mind-set, 186, 196–200
    learning to quiet, as facet of
    supersexual mind-set,
    186, 187–188
Mind-set, supersexual, facets
    of, 186–207
"Miracles" (Whitman), 198
Mysticism, supersex and,
    20–25
Myths of satisfying sex, 16–17

Neurosis and Human Growth (Horney), 94
Novelty, as myth in satisfying sex, 17

Once Upon a Midlife (Chinen), 114
Oneness, sense of, supersex and, 48–50, 64–67
Openness, feeling of
peak experience and, 62
as facet of supersexual mindset, 186
Ordinary People as Monks and Mystics (Sinetar), 112
Orgasm
and altered state of consciousness, 24–25
genitally focused, as myth of satisfying sex, 17, 25
lack of, in unsatisfying sex, 8
"no hands," 147
supersex and, 27–28

Pain
as problem in unsatisfying sex, 8
and sudden supersexual transformation, 128
Parents, effect of, on supersexual women, 108–111
Partner
role of, in supersex, 79–92
trust of, as facet of supersexual mind-set, 186, 190–193

"wrong," supersex with, 43–44
Passages (Sheehy), 107
Past, vividly re-experiencing (Cluster 4), 146
Patience, as characteristic of supersexual women, 132–134
Peak experience, 23–24, 61–64
dimensions of, 62
supersex and, 64
See also Ecstasy, supersexual
Peak performance vs. supersex, 56–58
Peak sex. *See* Supersex
Performance, peak, vs. supersex, 56–58
Perls, Fritz, 50
Physical endowment, importance of, as myth of satisfactory sex, 17
Porizkova, Paulina, 84
Privette, Gayle, 58
Psychobiology of Consciousness, The (Davidson), 24
Psychology, Gestalt, 50

Reich, Wilhelm, 201
Relationships
effect on, of supersex, 90–92
I-It, 75
I-Thou, 74–77, 149
Relaxation Response (Benson), 188
Religion
supersex and, 22

246

Index

supersexual women and,
102–103
see also specific religions
Respect, feeling of, supersex
and, 86–87
"Rightness," sense of,
supersex and, 51

*Sacred Sexuality: Living the
Vision of the Erotic
Spirit* (Feuerstein), 28
Safety, feeling of, supersex
and, 51–52, 82–83
Schopenhauer, Arthur, 63
Self
limiting, vs. true self, and
sexuality, 95–96
true
contact with, to achieve
supersex, 94–95
contact with, as
characteristic of
supersexual women,
102
limiting self vs., and
sexuality, 95–96
trust of, as facet of
supersexual mind-set,
186, 190–193
Self-consciousness,
disappearance of,
supersex and, 46–47,
60–61
Self-empowerment
as characteristic of
supersexual women,
99–101
as factor in achieving
supersex, 100–101

"Self-forgetting," supersex
and, 47–48
Self-knowing, supersex and,
116, 121
Senses, enhancing enjoyment
of, as facet of
supersexual mind-set,
186, 200–207,
Serenity Prayer, 119–120
Sex
satisfying
factors in, 8
myths of, 16–17
unsatisfying, problems of, 8
see also Sexuality; Supersex
Sexuality
attitudes about, and choices
in love, 194–196
limiting self vs. true self
and, 95–96
see also Sex; Supersex
Shakespeare, William, 201
Sheehy, Gail, 107
Siebert, Al, 100–101
Siegel, Dr. Bernie, 101
Silent Pulse, The (Leonard),
56
Sinetar, Marsha, 112–113
Smells, as manifestation of
supersexual ecstasy,
20, 148
Solitude, effect of, on
supersexual women,
111–113
Sounds, as manifestation of
supersexual ecstasy, 7,
148
Spiritual connection (Cluster
7), 149–150

Spontaneity, supersex and,
121
Staying connected to thing
loved, as facet of
supersexual mind-set,
186, 188–190
Stock, Wendy E., 116
Straining, lack of, as
dimension of peak
experience, 62
Supersex
as altered state of
consciousness, 24–25
and disappearance of self-
consciousness, 46–47,
60–61
effect of, on relationships,
90–92
and feeling of safety, 51–52,
82–83
and flow, 59–61
means of achieving, 93–104
and meditation, 187–88
and mysticism, 20–25
orgasm and, 27–28
and peak experience, 64
vs. peak performance,
56–58
post-divorce, 40–43
potential for, quiz on,
138–141
and relaxed concentration,
50
and religion, 22
role of partner in, 79–92
and "self-forgetting," 47–48
and self-knowing, 116, 121
and sense of
connectedness, 64–67
and sense of "knowing,"
52–54
and sense of oneness,
48–50, 64–67
and sense of "rightness," 51
studies in, 25–30
sudden awakening to,
causes of, 128
term defined, 8–9
as timeless state, 45–46, 56
with "wrong" partner,
43–44
Supersexual ecstasy. *See*
Ecstasy, supersexual
Supersexual mind-set. *See*
Mind-set, supersexual
"Survivors"
characteristics of, 100–101
supersexual women as,
100–101

Tantric Hinduism, mysticism
and sex in, 24–25, 30
Taoism, mysticism and sex in,
24–25
Tao of Physics, The (Capra), 63
Tellegen, Auke, 10
Tellegen scale, 10, 142
Thich Nhat Hanh, 187–188
Timeless state, supersex as,
45–46, 56
Tolkien, J.R.R., 113–114
"True" voice, finding, as facet
of supersexual mind-
set, 186, 193–196
Trust
as factor in supersex, 80, 85
and supersexual mind-set,
186, 190–193

Upanishads (religious text),
     63

Vance, Ellen Belle, Ph.D.,
     27
Visions, as manifestation of
     sexual ecstasy, 7,
     19–20, 28, 29, 32–33
Voice, "true," finding, as facet
     of supersexual mind-
     set, 186, 193–196

Wagner, Nathaniel N., Ph.D.,
     27
Whitman, Walt, 198

Wisdom, inner, supersex and,
     128–132
Women, supersexual
     characteristics of, 100–104,
     132–134
     effect on, of parents,
     108–111
     and religion, 102–103
     as "survivors," 100–101
     young, characteristics of,
     107–116
Wordsworth, William, 35

Zorba the Greek (Kazantzakis),
     132–133